Temple Ritual & Theater & Drama

Of the

Ancient Egyptian

Mysteries

Including the Ancient Egyptian Play

The Enlightenment Of Hetheru
By
Muata Ashby

©1998-2002

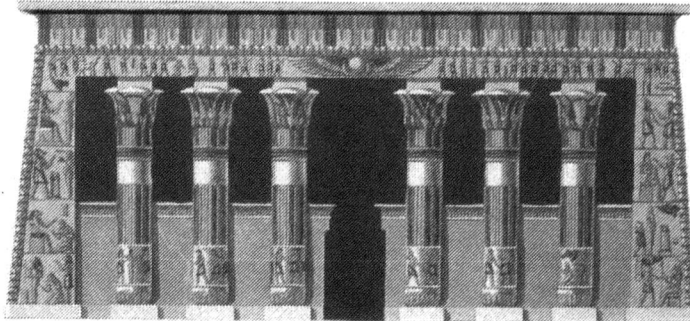

Sema
Institute of Yoga

Sema (☥) is an ancient Egyptian word and symbol meaning *union*. The Sema Institute is dedicated to the propagation of the universal teachings of spiritual evolution which relate to the union of humanity and the union of all things within the universe. It is a non-denominational organization which recognizes the unifying principles in all spiritual and religious systems of evolution throughout the world. Our primary goals are to provide the wisdom of ancient spiritual teachings in books, courses and other forms of communication. Secondly, to provide expert instruction and training in the various yogic disciplines including Ancient Egyptian Philosophy, Christian Gnosticism, Indian Philosophy and modern science. Thirdly, to promote world peace and Universal Love.

A primary focus of our tradition is to identify and acknowledge the yogic principles within all religions and to relate them to each other in order to promote their deeper understanding as well as to show the essential unity of purpose and the unity of all living beings and nature within the whole of existence.

The Institute is open to all who believe in the principles of peace, non-violence and spiritual emancipation regardless of sex, race, or creed.

Sema Institute
P.O. Box 570459, Miami, Fla. 33257 (305) 378-6253,
Fax (305) 378-6253
©1997-2005

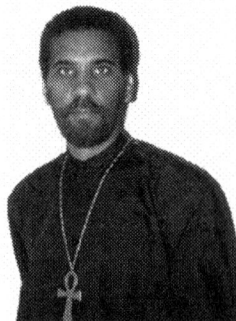

About the author and editor:

About The Author

Reginald Muata Ashby holds a Doctor of Philosophy Degree in Religion, and a Doctor of Divinity Degree in Holistic Healing. He is also a Pastoral Counselor and Teacher of Yoga Philosophy and Discipline. Dr. Ashby is an adjunct faculty member of the American Institute of Holistic Theology and an ordained Minister. Dr. Ashby has studied advanced Jnana, Bhakti and Kundalini Yogas under the guidance of Swami Jyotirmayananda, a world renowned Yoga Master. He has studied the mystical teachings of ancient Egypt for many years and is the creator of the Egyptian Yoga concept. He is also the founder of the Sema Institute, an organization dedicated to the propagation of the teachings of Yoga and mystical spirituality.

Dr. Ashby began his research into the spiritual philosophy of Ancient Africa (Egypt) and India and noticed correlations in the culture and arts of the two countries. This was the catalyst for a successful book series on the subject called "Egyptian Yoga". Now he has created a series of musical compositions which explore this unique area of music from ancient Egypt and its connection to world music.

Karen Clarke-Ashby "Dja" is the wife and spiritual partner of Muata. She is an independent researcher, practitioner and certified teacher of Yoga, a Doctor in the Sciences and a Pastoral Counselor, the editor of Egyptian Proverbs and Egyptian Yoga by Muata.☥

Cruzian Mystic Books/Sema Institute of Yoga
P.O.Box 570459
Miami, Florida, 33257
(305) 378-6253 Fax: (305) 378-6253

© 1998-2002-2006

By Reginald Muata Abhaya Ashby

The author is available for group lectures and individual counseling. For further information contact the publisher.

Ashby, Muata
The Enlightenment of Hetheru ISBN: 1-884564-14-3

Library of Congress Cataloging in Publication Data

1 Ancient Egyptian Theater, 2 Egyptian Mythology 3 Spirituality 4 Religion 5 Yoga 6 Self Help.

Table of Contents

About Ancient Egypt:

"Ancient KMT is the Image of Heaven and the
Shrine of the World."

"KMT"
"Egypt", "Burnt", "Land of Blackness", "Land of the Burnt People."

"India taken as a whole, beginning from the north and embracing what of it is subject to Persia, is a continuation of Egypt and the Ethiopians."

The Itinerarium Alexandri   A.C.E. 345

"There are Egyptian columns as far off as NYASA, Arabia...Aset and Asar led an army into India, to the source of the Ganges, and as far as the Indus Ocean."

Recorded by Egyptian High Priest *Manetho* (300 B.C.) and
***Diodorus* (Greek historian 100 B. C.)**

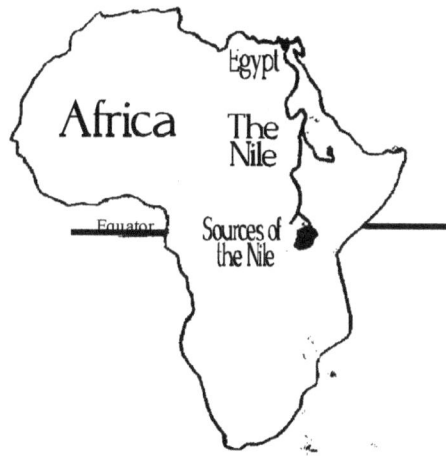

ABOUT THE ANCIENT EGYPTIANS:

"Our people originated at the base of the mountain of the Moon, at the origin of the Nile river."†

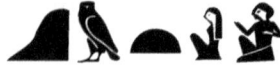

"They also say that the Egyptians are colonists sent out by the Ethiopians, Asar having been the leader of the colony."

-Diodorus Siculus

"When therefore, you hear the myths of the Egyptians concerning the Gods - wanderings and dismemberings and many such passions, think none of these things spoken as they really are in state and action. For they do not call Hermes "Dog" as a proper name, but they associate the watching and waking from sleep of the animal who by Knowing and not Knowing determines friend from foe with the most Logos-like of the Gods."

-Plutarch

"The Egyptians and Nubians have thick lips, broad noses, woolly hair and burnt skin...
...And the Indian tribes I have mentioned, their skins are all of the same color, much like the Ethiopians... their country is a long way from Persia towards the south..."

- Herodotus

"The riches of Egypt are for the foreigners therein."

-Anonymous Arabic proverb.

"Truly at weaving wiles the Egyptians are clever."

-Anonymous

The Ethiopians and Egyptians are very black."

- Aristotle

"Compared with the Egyptians, the Greeks are childish mathematicians."

- Plato

"And upon his return to Greece, they gathered around and asked, "tell us about this great land of the Blacks called Ethiopia." And Herodotus said, "There are two great Ethiopian nations, one in Sind (India) and the other in Egypt."

- Recorded by Diodorus (Greek historian 100 B.C.)

The Term Kamit (Qamit, Kamit, Kamit) and Its Relation to Nubia and the term "Black"

As we have seen, the terms "Ethiopia," "Nubia," "Kush" and "Sudan" all refer to "black land" and/or the "land of the blacks." In the same manner we find that the name of Egypt which was used by the Ancient Egyptians also means "black land" and/or the "land of the blacks." The hieroglyphs below reveal the Ancient Egyptian meaning of the words related to the name of their land. It is clear that the meaning of the word Qamit is equivalent to the word Kush as far as they relate to "black land" and that they also refer to a differentiation in geographical location, i.e. Kush is the "black land of the south" and Qamit is the "black land of the north." Both terms denote the primary quality that defines Africa, "black" or "Blackness" (referring to the land and its people). The quality of blackness and the consonantal sound of K or Q as well as the reference to the land are all aspects of commonality between the Ancient Kushitic and Kamitan terms.

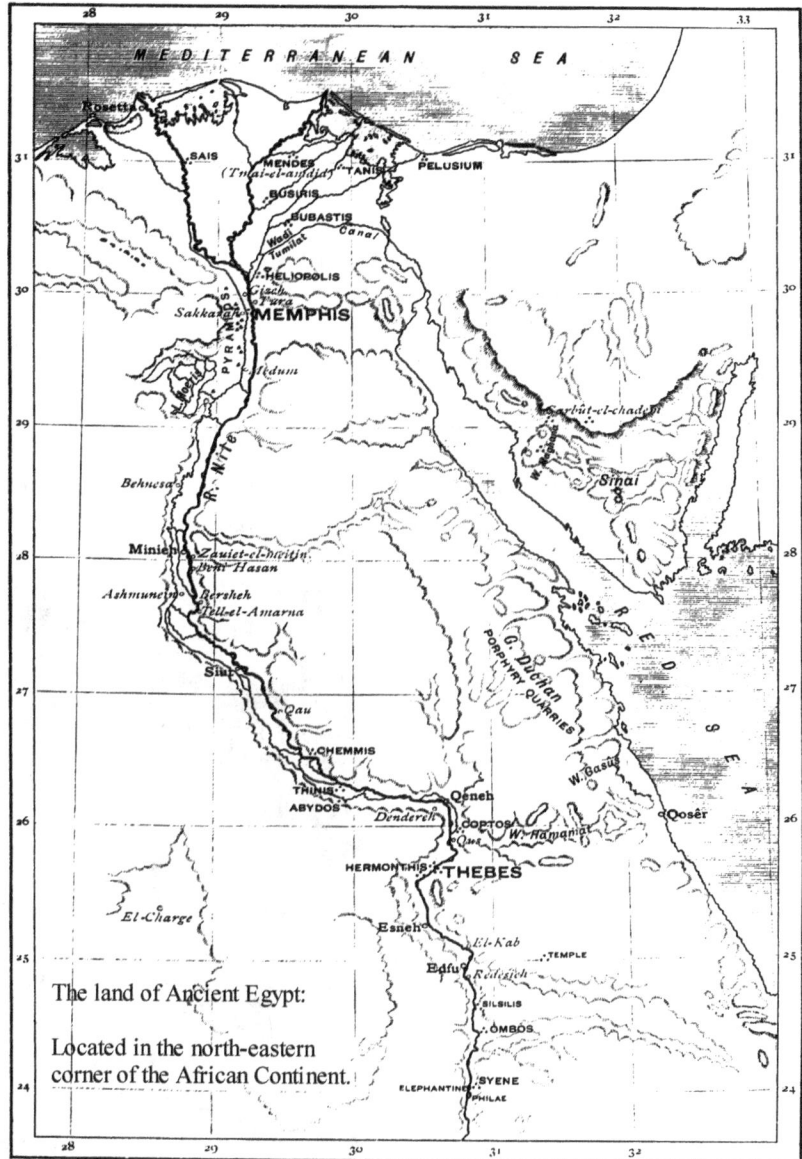

The land of Ancient Egypt:

Located in the north-eastern corner of the African Continent.

Qamit - Ancient Egypt.

Qamit - blackness – black.

Qamit - literature of Ancient Egypt – scriptures.

9

Qamiu or variant - Ancient Egyptians-people of the black land.

A Long History

For a period spanning over 10,000 years the Neterian religion served the society of ancient Kamit. It is hard to comprehend the vastness of time that is encompassed by Ancient Egyptian culture, religion and philosophy. Yet the evidence is there to be seen by all. It has been collected and presented in the book *African Origins of Civilization, Religion and Yoga Philosophy.* That volume will serve as the historical record for the Neterian religion and as record of its legacy to all humanity. It serves as the basis or foundation for the work contained in all the other books in this series that have been created to elucidate on the teachings and traditions as well as disciplines of the varied Neterian religious traditions.

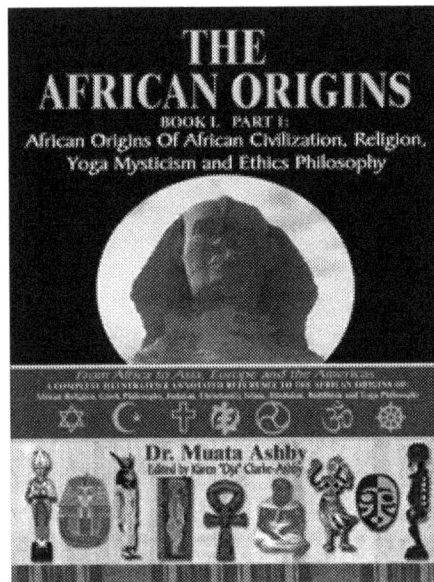

The book *African Origins of Civilization, Religion and Yoga Philosophy,* and the other volumes on the specific traditions detail the philosophies and disciplines that should be practiced by those who want to follow the path of Hm or Hmt, to be practitioners of the Shetaut Neter religion and builders of the Neterian faith worldwide.

Many people often ask why Ancient Egyptian culture and society deteriorated. The following excerpt from the book *African Origins of Civilization, Religion and Yoga Philosophy,* presents some of the most important causative factors for the decline. However, central among these are the minimization of the Hemu (clergy) and the turn away from Maat (righteousness) in government, and cultural values.

The Ancient Egyptian religion (*Shetaut Neter*), language and symbols provide the first "historical" record of Yoga Philosophy and Religious literature. Egyptian Yoga is what has been commonly referred to by Egyptologists as Egyptian "Religion" or "Mythology", but to think of it as just another set of stories or allegories about a long lost civilization is to completely miss the greatest secret of human existence. Yoga, in all of its forms and disciplines of spiritual development, was practiced in Egypt earlier than anywhere else in history. This unique perspective from the highest philosophical system which developed in Africa over seven thousand years ago provides a new way to look at life, religion, the discipline of psychology and the way to spiritual development leading to spiritual Enlightenment. Egyptian mythology, when understood as a system of Yoga (union of the individual soul with the Universal Soul or Supreme Consciousness), gives every individual insight into their own divine nature and also a deeper insight into all religions and Yoga systems.

Who Were the Ancient Egyptians and What is Yoga Philosophy?

Diodorus Siculus (Greek Historian) writes in the time of Augustus (first century B.C.):

"Now the Ethiopians, as historians relate, were the first of all men and the proofs of this statement, they say, are manifest. For that they did not come into their land as immigrants from abroad but were the natives of it and so justly bear the name of autochthones (sprung from the soil itself), is, they maintain, conceded by practically all men..."

"They also say that the Egyptians are colonists sent out by the Ethiopians, Asar having been the leader of the colony. For, speaking generally, what is now Egypt, they maintain, was not land, but sea, when in the beginning the universe was being formed; afterwards, however, as the Nile during the times of its inundation carried down the mud from Ethiopia, land was gradually built up from the deposit...And the larger parts of the customs of the Egyptians are, they hold, Ethiopian, the colonists still preserving their ancient manners. For instance, the belief that their kings are Gods, the very special attention which they pay to their burials, and many other matters of a similar nature, are Ethiopian practices, while the shapes of their statues and the forms of their letters are Ethiopian; for of the two kinds of writing which the Egyptians have, that which is known as popular (demotic) is learned by everyone, while that which is called sacred (hieratic), is understood only by the priests of the Egyptians, who learnt it from their Fathers as one of the things which are not divulged, but among the Ethiopians, everyone uses these forms of letters. Furthermore, the orders of the priests, they maintain, have much the same position among both peoples; for all are clean who are engaged in the service of the gods, keeping themselves shaven, like the Ethiopian priests, and having the same dress and form of staff, which is shaped like a plough and is carried by their kings who wear high felt hats which end in a knob in the top and are circled by the serpents which they call asps; and this symbol appears to carry the thought that it will be the lot who shall dare to attack the king to encounter death-carrying stings. Many other things are told by them concerning their own antiquity and the colony which they sent out that became the Egyptians, but about this there is no special need of our writing anything."

The Ancient Egyptian texts state:

"Our people originated at the base of the mountain of the Moon,

at the origin of the Nile river."

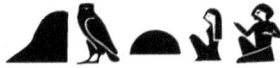

"KMT" "Egypt", "Burnt", "Land of Blackness","Land of the Burnt People."

KMT (Ancient Egypt) is situated close to Lake Victoria in present day Africa. This is the same location where the earliest human remains have been found, in the land currently known as Ethiopia-Tanzania. Recent genetic technology as reported in the new encyclopedias and leading news publications has revealed that all peoples of the world originated in Africa and migrated to other parts of the world prior to the last Ice Age 40,000 years ago. Therefore, as of this time, genetic testing has revealed that all humans are alike. The earliest bone fossils which have been found in many parts of the world were those of the African Grimaldi type. During the Ice Age, it was not possible to communicate or to migrate. Those trapped in specific locations were subject to the regional forces of weather and climate. Less warmer climates required less body pigment, thereby producing lighter pigmented people who now differed from their dark-skinned ancestors. After the Ice Age when travel was possible, these light-skinned people who had lived in the northern, colder regions of harsh weather during the Ice Age period moved back to the warmer climates of their ancestors, and mixed with the people there who had remained dark-skinned, thereby producing the Semitic colored people. "Semite" means mixture of skin color shades.

Therefore, there is only one human race who, due to different climactic and regional exposure, changed to a point where there seemed to be different "types" of people. Differences were noted with respect to skin color, hair texture, customs, languages, and with respect to the essential nature (psychological and emotional makeup) due to the experiences each group had to face and overcome in order to survive.

From a philosophical standpoint, the question as to the origin of humanity is redundant when it is understood that _ALL_ come from one origin which some choose to call the "Big Bang" and others "The Supreme Being."

> **"Thou makest the color of the skin of one race to be different from that of another, but however many may be the varieties of mankind, it is thou that makes them all to live."**
> —Ancient Egyptian Proverb from *The Hymns of Amun*

> **"Souls, Heru, son, are of the self-same nature, since they came from the same place where the Creator modeled them; nor male nor female are they. Sex is a thing of bodies not of Souls."**
> —Ancient Egyptian Proverb from *The teachings of Aset to Heru*

Historical evidence proves that Ethiopia-Nubia already had Kingdoms at least 300 years before the first Kingdom-Pharaoh of Egypt.

> ***"Ancient Egypt was a colony of Nubia - Ethiopia. ...Asar having been the leader of the colony..."***

"And upon his return to Greece, they gathered around and asked, "tell us about this great land of the Blacks called Ethiopia." And Herodotus said, "There are two great Ethiopian nations, one in Sind (India) and the other in Egypt."

**Recorded by Egyptian high priest *Manetho* (300 B.C.)
also Recorded by *Diodorus* (Greek historian 100 B.C.)**

The pyramids themselves however, cannot be dated, but indications are that they existed far back in antiquity. The Pyramid Texts (hieroglyphics inscribed on pyramid walls) and Coffin Texts (hieroglyphics inscribed on coffins) speak authoritatively on the constitution of the human spirit, the vital Life Force along the human spinal cord (known in India as *"Kundalini"*), the immortality of the soul, reincarnation and the law of Cause and Effect (known in India as the Law of Karma).

Below- Ancient Egyptian man and woman-(tomb of Payry) 18th Dynasty displaying the naturalistic style (as people really appeared in ancient times).

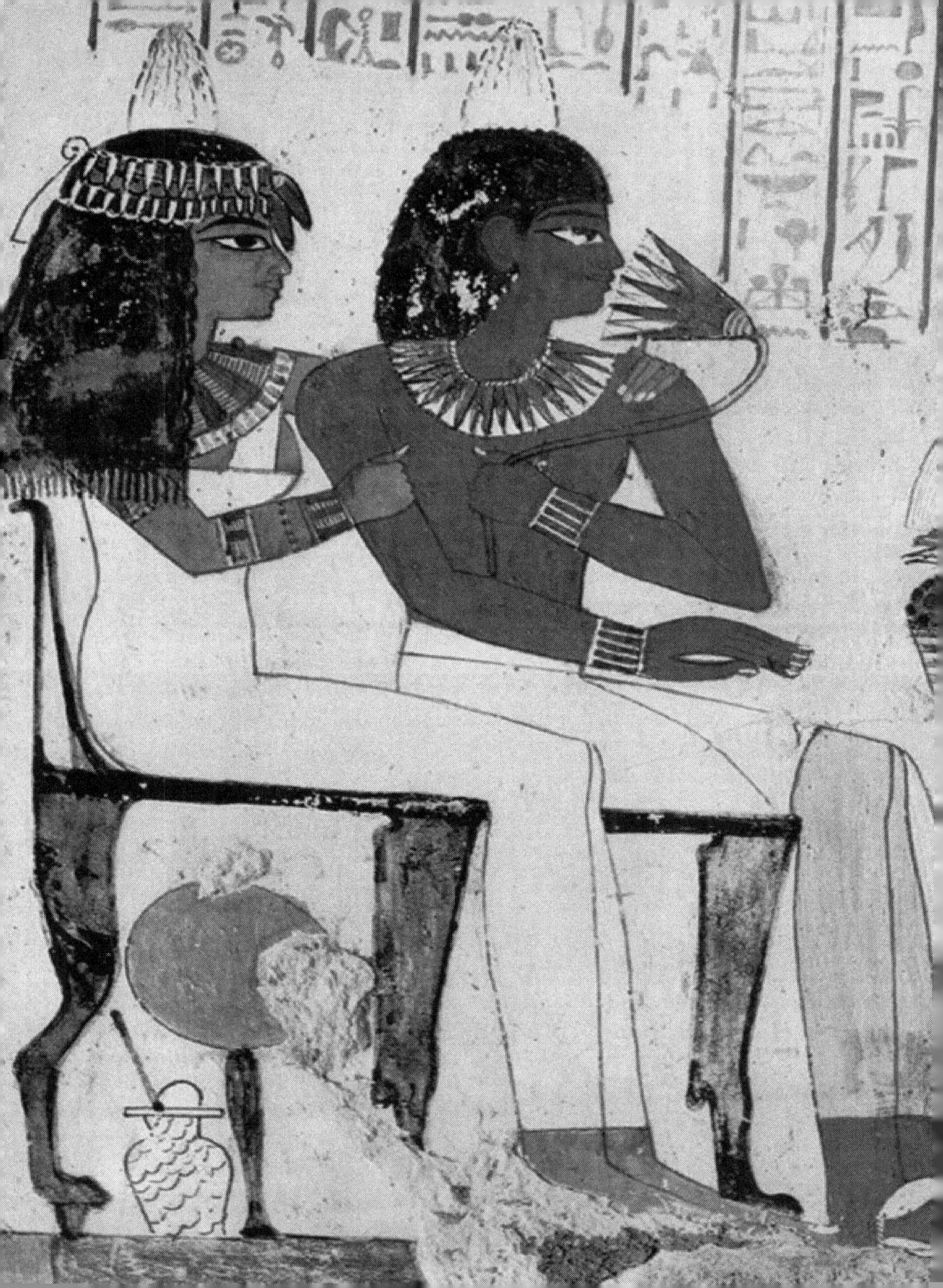

What is Shetaut Neter?

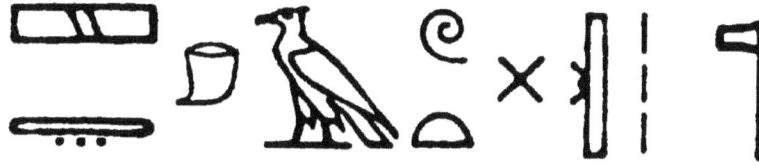

Goddess worship is one branch of Shetaut Neter. Shetaut Neter is the name that the ancient African (Egyptians) gave to their religion. The Ancient Egyptians were African peoples who lived in the north-eastern quadrant of the continent of Africa. They were descendants of the Nubians, who had themselves originated from farther south into the heart of Africa at the great lakes region, the sources of the Nile River. They created a vast civilization and culture earlier than any other society in known history and organized a nation which was based on the concepts of balance and order as well as spiritual enlightenment. These ancient African people called their land Kamit and soon after developing a well ordered society they began to realize that the world is full of wonders but life is fleeting and that there must be something more to human existence. They developed spiritual systems that were designed to allow human beings to understand the nature of this secret being who is the essence of all Creation. They called this spiritual system "Shtaut Ntr."

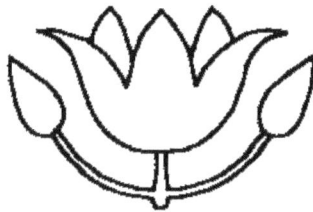

The Spiritual Culture and the Purpose of Life: Shetaut Neter

The highest forms of Joy, Peace and Contentment are obtained when the meaning of life is discovered. When the human being is in harmony then it is possible to reflect and meditate upon the human condition and realize the limitations of worldly pursuits. When there is peace and harmony a human being can practice any of the varied disciplines, designated as Shetaut Neter, to promote the evolution of the human being towards the ultimate goal of life which Spiritual Enlightenment. Spiritual Enlightenment is the awakening of the human being to the awareness of the transcendental essence which binds the universe and which is eternal and immutable. In this discovery is also the sobering and ecstatic realization that the human being is one with that transcendental essence. With this realization come great joy, peace and power to experience the fullness of live and to realize the purpose of life during the time on earth. The lotus is a symbol of Shetaut Neter, meaning the turning towards the light of truth, peace and transcendental harmony.

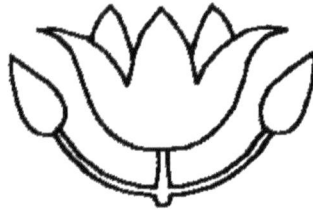

FOREWORD

Temple reenactments of the myths was a prominent and integral aspect of Neterian (Ancient Egyptian) religion. Assuming the role of a divinity allows the participant to come closer to the divinities and to thereby understand him/her self better and attain enlightenment. The most prominent and important plays in Neterian religion were

1. The passion of Asar
2. The Divine Cow (Enlightenment of Hetheru or The Story of Hetheru and Djehuti)
3. Contendings of Heru and Set
4. The Creation Myth

Thus, in order to properly understand the religion of Ancient Egypt it is also necessary to understand the drama of the Temple Mysteries and conversely, in order to understand the Temple Mysteries it is necessary to understand the Temple Theater. And in order to understand the Temple Theater it is necessary to actually act out the drama of the myth in question. This act allows the participant to gain an insight into the mysteries that is otherwise impossible. Thus, the temple rituals of Ancient Egypt were at the same time drama, reenactment, role-playing and identification of the individual with the Divine, the Higher Self.

I am very happy to have the opportunity to bring forth this wonderful drama from Ancient Egypt which is timeless in nature. The reader may note certain similarities to modern dramas which have been brought to the movie screens and to Broadway as well, namely, "The Lion King." Whether or not the writers of The Lion King knew of the similarities it shares with the "The Enlightenment of Hetheru," is for the reader to judge.

It is clear however that Ancient Egyptian culture has had and continues to have an effect on modern society. This timeless story, "The Enlightenment of Hetheru," epitomizes the Ancient Egyptian concept of mythology which links the Divine to human beings, for it was said in ancient times that Hetheru's (Hathor's) journey is in reality the journey of every human being. We all come into the world and get lost in the wilderness of life and eventually someone comes along to help us in various ways.

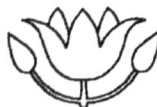

HISTORICAL BACKGROUND OF ANCIENT EGYPTIAN THEATER

Definition and Origin of: "Theater"

> **A place or building in which dramatic performances for an audience take place; these include drama, dancing, music, mime, opera, ballet, and puppets.**
>
> **Theatre history can be traced to (Ancient) Egyptian religious ritualistic drama as long ago as 3200 BC. The first known European theaters were in Greece from about 600 BC.**
>
> -Copyright © 1995 Websters Encyclopedia
> Helicon Publishing Ltd.

Many people believe that the art of theater began with the ancient Greek theater. Thespis, the first actor-dramatist (about 560 B.C.E.), is considered to have been the first person to give the Greek drama its form; actors are still called "thespians." However, upon closer examination, it must be noted that just as Greek philosophers such as Thales and Pythagoras learned their wisdom from the Ancient Egyptians and then set up their schools of philosophy in Greece, it is likely that the first Greek actors and playwrights learned their profession from the Ancient Egyptian Sages when they came from Greece to learn the religion and the sciences.[1] Actually, a great debt is owed to the Greek writers of ancient times because their records attest to many details which the Ancient Egyptians did not record.

Ancient Greek theater had its origin in the mysteries of Dionysus. It is well known to scholars of Ancient Greece and Greek mythology that Orpheus is credited with introducing the cult of Dionysus to Greece along with its initiatory rites.

> Orpheus, king of the <u>Ciconians</u>, is counted among the <u>ARGONAUTS</u>. Orpheus practiced minstrelsy and by his songs moved stones and trees, holding also a spell over the wild beasts. He descended to the <u>Underworld</u> in order to fetch his dead wife, but had to return without her. Orpheus, whom <u>Apollo</u> taught to play the lyre, traveled to Egypt where he increased his knowledge about the gods and their initiatory rites, bringing from that country most of his mystic ceremonies, orgiastic rites, and his extraordinary account of his descent to the <u>Underworld</u>. Orpheus became famous because of his poems and his songs, excelling everyone in the beauty of his verse and music. He also reached a high degree of influence because he was believed to have discovered mysteries, purification from sins, cures of diseases, and means of averting divine wrath. Some say that Orpheus introduced a cult of <u>Dionysus 2</u> that was very similar to the cult of Osiris, and that

---

[1] see the book "From Egypt to Greece" by Muata Ashby available through the Sema Institute and bookstores.

of Isis, which resembles the cult of Demeter. But others affirm that he praised all the gods except Dionysus 2.[2]

Upon cursory investigation it is discovered that Dionysus is the Greeks name for the god Asar (Osiris). The Greek writings attest to the fact the Dionysus was the same Osiris, brought into Greece from Egypt. The dates of the prominence of Dionysus coincide with the association of the first Greek philosophers of the Greek classical period with the Ancient Egyptian priests. The qualities of Dionysus are the same as those of the Egyptian Asar and the temple mysteries including vegetation, death and resurrection, were also the same. The enactment of those mysteries constitutes the Egyptian "Theater" which was adopted by the Greeks and which was later developed by the Greek playwrights into other themes.[3] (highlighted text by Ashby)

> Born of the union of Zeus and a mortal, Semele, **Dionysos rose to prominence around the 6th century B.C. under many names and forms.** The principles of life and generation, as well as the cyclical life of vegetation (death and rebirth), are central to the worship of Dionysos: lord of the vine, but also god of the tree. He is often considered in reference to the fig tree, ivy (undying life), and all blossoming things -- symbols of life and vitality. His celebration is marked by the joy of his epiphany in the Spring, and the sorrow of his death or descent in the Winter. Dionysos also appears as a bull god, long considered an important symbol of fertility in the Ancient World. Other symbols that are associated with him include snakes, goats, lightening bolts, as well as moistness, madness and the phallus. Dionysos is typically followed by satyrs and maenads who participate in the music, wine, and dancing which make up an integral aspect of his mystery. Satyrs, or primitive, goat-like men, usually lurk in the shadows of the more primary maenads, or mad women, which typified Dionysian worship. These maenads, "the frenzied sanctified women who are devoted to the worship of Dionysos."(Harrison -401), are 'nurses' who look after and follow the infant Dionysos-- likely referring to the largely female following he inspired and the great Mother goddess he came from.[4]

This section has been included to show the importance of theatrical-ritual in Neterian spirituality. It must be clear though that this form of art is reserved for the realm of spirituality and not for frivolous entertainment.

---

[2] *Greek Mythology Link*, created and maintained by Carlos Parada. Since 1997© 1993-2004 http://homepage.mac.com/cparada/GML/index.html

[3] Origin of the Greek Theater by B. H. Stricker, Journal of Egyptian Archeology

[4] *Greek Mythology Link*, created and maintained by Carlos Parada. Since 1997© 1993-2004 http://homepage.mac.com/cparada/GML/index.html

The African Origins of The Greek God Dionysus and the Ancient Egyptian Origins of Ancient Greek Theater in the Mysteries of Dionysus

The ancient Greeks themselves documented that their main gods and goddesses came from Ancient Egypt. Asar was one of the most important gods of Ancient Egypt and similarly as well in ancient Greece under the name Dionysus. However, the mysteries of Asar, though including the concept of festivity, were exaggerated in the Greek adoption in the aspect of the god as being the god of wine, pleasure, etc.

The following image is of a Black figured vase. The Black figured vases are ancient Greek vases with black figures painted on reddish orange clay. In the Black figured vases the details within the silhouetted figures were incised before firing. The following image contains the god Dionysus and the Maenads.

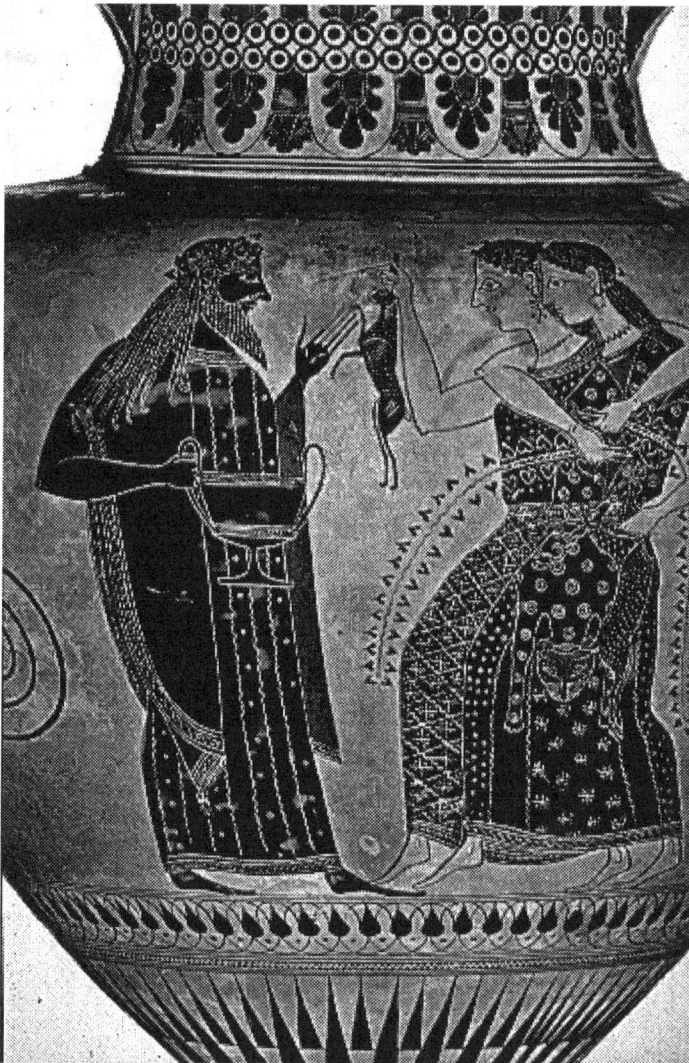

The following description of the vase was given by Loggia Art:
This beautiful black figure vase painting by the Amasis Painter depicts Dionysos with a pair of attendant maenads. The image appears on a type of vessel that the ancient Greeks called an amphora. Amphorae (the plural form of the word amphora) were used to store such treasures as wine and oil.
The body of the vase is adorned with a gorgeous group of figures. Dionysos, the Greek god of wine and the theatre, stands on the left. The god is bearded and holds a kantharos (this kind of wine cup is often used as a symbol of Dionysos) in one of his hands. The right side of the vase features two women, who are often identified as maenads (female followers of Dionysos). These women are intertwined and clad in dark, intricately detailed garments. One of the maenads is holding a hare, while the other is carrying a deer. Each of the female figures is also grasping a sprig of stylized ivy. Notice how the skin of the male figure - Dionysos - is dark, while the female figures - the maenads - both have pale, buff colored skin. [1]

---

[5] http://www.usc.edu/dept/finearts/slide/pollini/Lecture6.html/250.html

Notice that the top and bottom of the vase has classical lotus symbols of the ancient Egyptian Lotus. Further, the symbol of the hare is one of the primary signs of the Ancient Egyptian God Asar (Osiris). In fact, one of the main titles of Asar is "Unefer"

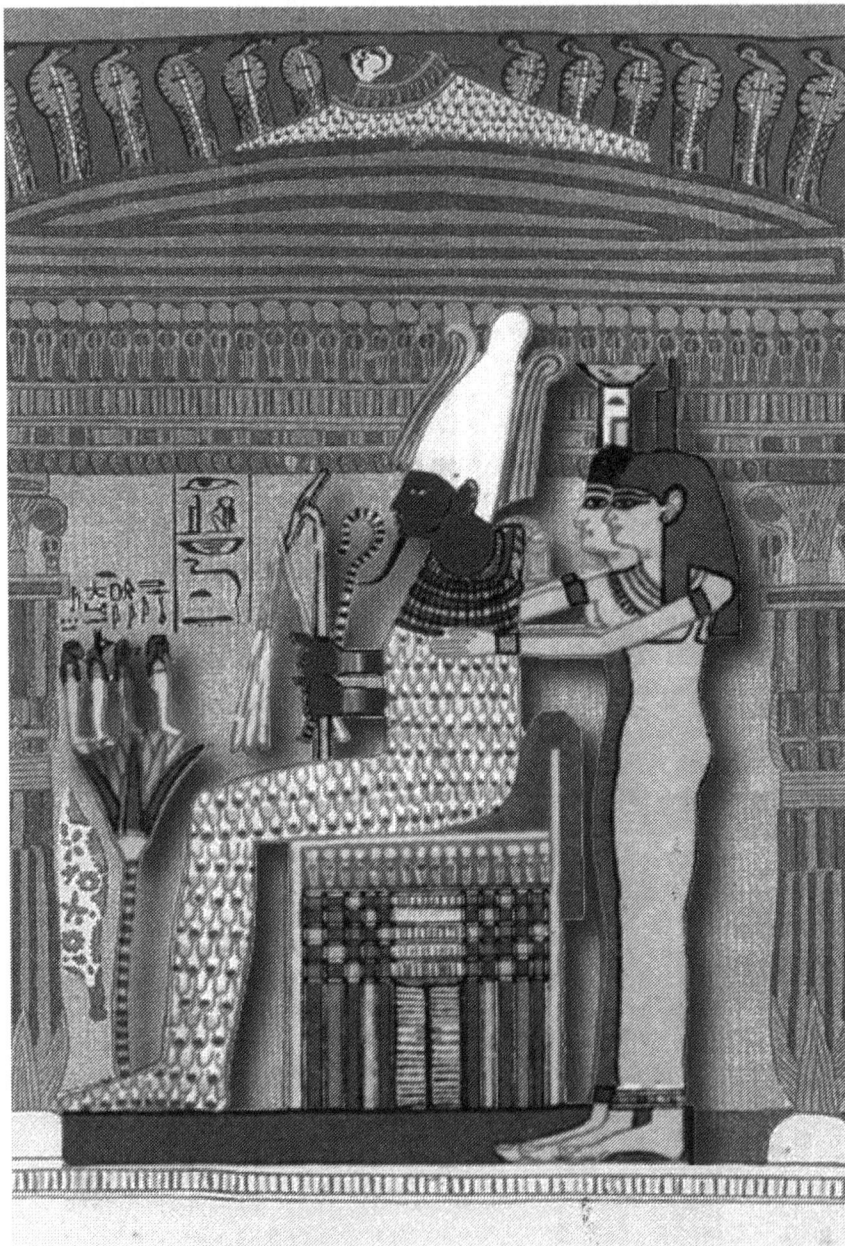

NOTE: the similarity in the black hue of Dionysus and his female companionship with white hue in the Greek iconography of Dionysus and that odf Asar (Osiris).

The Ancient Egyptian God Asar is usually depicted with green or black hue and he is usually accompanied by the two female divinities Aset "Isis" and Nebethet "Nephthys".

The "two Ladies" are usually depicted as yellow or as white.

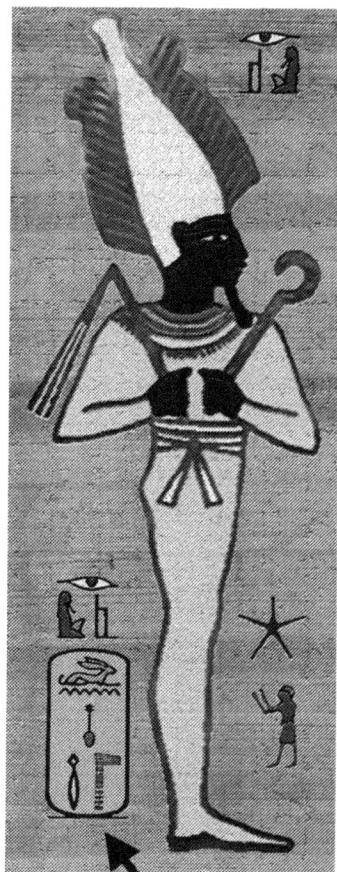

The Ancient Egyptian God Asar, depicted in black hue in his form as the "Lord of the Perfect Black"

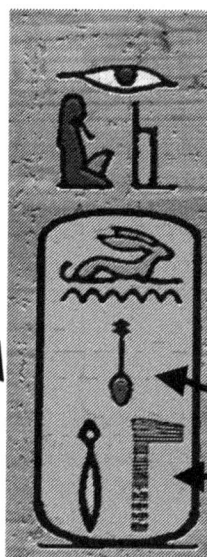

The name of Asar (the seeing one, the watching (seeing) consciousness).

Notice that the hare is used in Asar's main title:

Title:
"Un-Nefer Neter"
Un -singular
Nefer -beautiful
Neter existing-
Divinity Great)

The following excerpts from the book *History of Egypt* by Diodorus directly link the Ancient Egyptian god Asar (Osiris) with the Greek "Dionysus" as being one and the same. (Highlighted text by Ashby)

BOOK 1 II 1-5[6]

For when the names are translated into Greek Osiris means " many-eyed," and properly so; for in shedding his rays in every direction he surveys with many eyes, as it were, all land and sea. And the words of the poet I are also in agreement with this conception when he says:

The sun, who sees all things and hears all things.

And of the ancient Greek writers of mythology some give to Osiris the name Dionysus or, with a slight change in form, Sirius. One of them, Eumolpus, in his *Bacchic Hymn* speaks of Our Dionysus, shining like a star, With fiery eye in every ray; while Orpheus 2 Says:

NOTE: Greek mythology writers give the Greek name Dionysus to the Egyptian God Asar (Osiris) who is known as "firery eye." One of Asar's main symbols is the eye.

---

[6] *History of Egypt* by Diodorus

And this is why men call him Shining One And Dionysus.

BOOK 1. 12- 7-13. 2[7]

Now so far as the celestial gods are concerned whose genesis is from eternity, this is the account given by the Egyptians.

13. And besides these there are other gods, they say, who were terrestrial, having once been mortals, but who, by reason of their sagacity and the good services which they rendered to all men, attained immortality, some of them having even been kings in Egypt. Their names, when translated, are in some cases the same as those of the celestial gods, while others have a distinct appellation, such as

BOOK 1- 13. 2-14- 1

Helius, Cronus, and Rhea, and also the Zeus who is -alled Ammon by some, and besides these Hera and Hephaestus, also Hestia, and, finally, Hermes. Helius was the first king of the Egyptians, his name being the same as that of the heavenly star.' Some of the priests, however, say that Hephaestus was their first king, since he was the discoverer of fire and received the rule because of this service to mankind; for once, when a tree on the mountains had been struck by lightning and the forest near by was ablaze, Hephaestus went up to it, for it was winter-time and greatly enjoyed the beat; as the fire died down he kept adding fuel to it, and while keeping the fire going in this way he invited the rest of mankind to enjoy the advantage which came from it. Then Cronus became the ruler, and upon marrying his sister Rhea he begat Osiris and Isis, according to some writers of mythology, but, according to the majority, Zeus and Hera, whose high achievements gave them dominion over the entire universe. From these last were sprung five gods, one born on each of the five days which the Egyptians intercalate; 2 the names of these children were Osiris and Isis, and also Typhon, Apollo, and Aphrodite; and Osiris when translated is Dionysus, and Isis is more similar to Demeter than to any other goddess; and after Osiris married Isis and succeeded to the kingship he did many things of service to the social life of man.

> NOTE: The list of Divine rulers follows the same sequence as given in Anunian Theology of Ancient Egypt and the Ancient Egyptian account of Creation.

> "Osiris" translated is "Dionysus".

---

[7] *History of Egypt* **by Diodorus**

BOOK 1. 23. 1-5[8]

23. The number of years from Osiris and Isis, they say, to the reign of Alexander, who founded the city which bears his name in Egypt, is over ten thousand, but, according to other writers, a little less than twenty-three thousand. And those who say that the god 1 was born of Semele and Zeus in Boeotian Thebes are, according to the priests, simply inventing the tale. <u>For they say that Orpheus, upon visiting Egypt and participating in the initiation and mysteries of Dionysus, adopted them and as a favour to the descendants of Cadmus, since he was kindly disposed to them and received honours at their hands, transferred the birth of the god to Thebes; and the common people, partly out of ignorance and partly out of their desire to have the god thought to be a Greek, eagerly accepted his initiatory rites and mysteries.</u>

Orpheus was initiatied into the mysteries of Dionysus ("Asar" – Osiris) and brought that religion to Greece where it was adopted. He then said that the god was born in Thebes (Greece) to facilitate people's acceptance of it.

Table 1: Kamitan Names of the main Gods and Goddesses of Ancient Egypt and the Greek translation in common use.

Kamitan (Ancient Egyptian) Names	Greek Names
Amun	Zeus
Ra	Helios
Ptah	Hephastos
Nut	Rhea
Geb	Kronos
Net	Athena
Khonsu	Heracles
Set	Ares or Typhon
Bast	Artemis
Uadjit	Leto
Asar (Ausar)	Osiris or Hades
Aset (Auset)	Isis or Demeter
Nebthet	Nephthys
Anpu or Apuat	Anubis
Hetheru	Hathor (Aphrodite)
Heru	Horus or Apollo
Djehuti	Thoth or Hermes
Maat	Astraea or Themis
Ptah	Prometheus

---

[8] *History of Egypt* by **Diodorus**

Early Greek Playwrights

The Influence of Ancient Egyptian Philosophy and Theater on Greek playwrights, and the Roman and Christian Theater began through the influence of early Greek philosophers who had studied philosophy and the Temple Mysteries of Ancient Egypt. Thespis, who lived in the mid-6th century B.C.E., was the first known Greek poet, who, according to tradition, is the founder of drama. He is also credited with instituting the use of masks to disguise the performers. None of his works have survived.

Above: Ancient Greek Tragedy Mask

There are three important early Greek playwrights, many of whose works have survived and have influenced theater in Europe. Aeschylus (525-456 BC), Greek dramatist, was the earliest of the great tragic poets of Athens. He was the predecessor of Sophocles and Euripides and he called the father of Greek tragedy. From Herodotus, the best known historian of the time (484-425 B.C.E.), we learn of correspondences between the Ancient Egyptian gods and goddesses and the Greek gods and goddesses and also that Aeschylus drew from Ancient Egyptian myth and theater in his work.

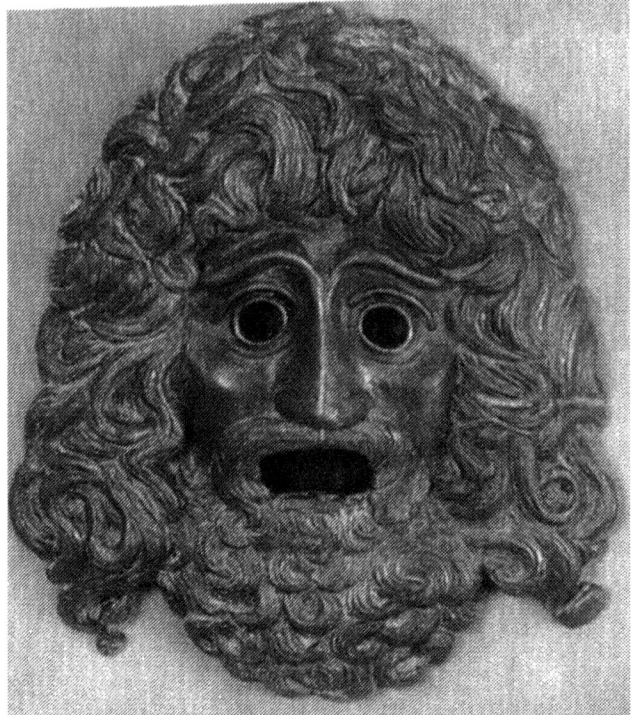

The Egyptians tell the following story in connection with this island, to explain the way in which it first came to float:- "In former times, when the isle was still fixed and motionless, Latona, one of the eight gods of the first order, who dwelt in the city of Buto, where now she has her oracle, received Apollo as a sacred charge from Isis, and saved him by hiding him in what is now called the floating island. Typhon meanwhile was searching everywhere in hopes of finding the child of Osiris."

(According to the Egyptians, Apollo and Diana are the children of Bacchus and Isis, while Latona is their nurse and their preserver. They call Apollo, in their language, Horus; Ceres they call Isis. From this Egyptian tradition, and from no other, it must have been that Aeschylus, the son of Euphorion, took the idea, which is found in none of the earlier poets, of making Diana the daughter of Ceres.) The island, therefore, in consequence of this event, was first made to float. Such at least is the account which the Egyptians give.

—Herodotus: The Histories (484-425 B.C.E.)

THE MIRACLE PLAY AND THE CHRISTIAN CHURCH

After the fall of Ancient Egyptian, Greek and Roman civilization, the Orthodox Christian church continued the practice of theater. There are many dramatic elements in the Roman Catholic services. Also, the use of theatrical techniques goes far back into the Church's history. In the Middle Ages, the services were popularized by the use of tableaux, of instructive pictures. Then the next step was to present the stories with live actors. The earliest religious play mentioned by name is the 'Play of St. Katherine.' It was produced in England in the 12th century.

During the 12th to the 14th centuries the plays moved from church control to secular actor's guilds and secular elements were added. The guilds went from street to street with large wagons, called pageants, on which they set up a stage with rude scenery . The Creation, Noah and the Flood, Adam and Eve, Abraham and Isaac, and other stories of the Old Testament were presented in addition to incidents in the life of Christ.

The mysteries presented stories from the Bible, and the miracle plays dealt with the lives of the saints. In association with these plays was another genre called moralities. In moralities, the moral lessons were taught by representing virtues and vices as persons. This form has been successfully revived in the 20th century.

Most of the plays originated as part of the religious teachings, but as they were taken over by the secular society they became corrupted by groups outside the clergy with vulgarities, witticisms and jests to the point that the church condemned them. They almost completely ceased to be performed after the 15th century. However, the Passion play can still be seen in modern church culture.

Masks of the Ancient Egyptian Theater

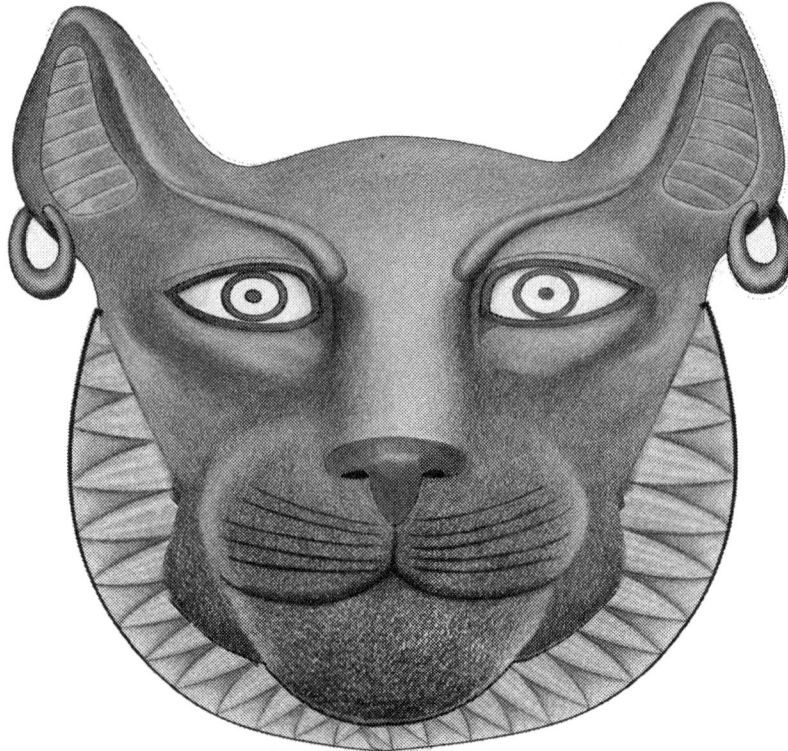

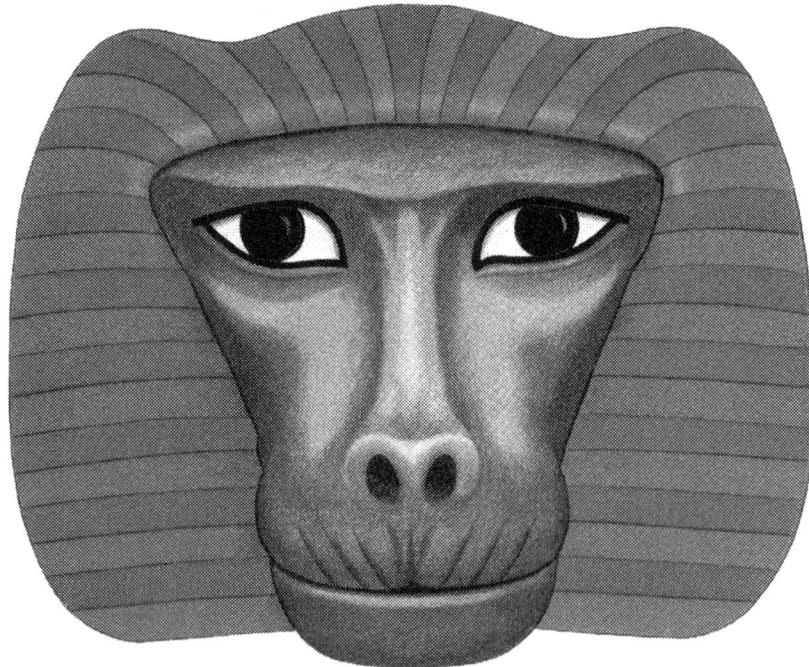

Above: Mask of the goddess Hetheru as a lioness.
Below: Mask of the god Djehuti as a baboon.

Euripides (circa 480-406 B.C.E.), was a Greek dramatist, the third, with Aeschylus and Sophocles, of the great Attic tragic poets. His work, fairly popular in his own time, exerted great influence on Roman drama. In more recent times he has influenced English and German drama, and most conspicuously, such French dramatic poets as Pierre Corneille and Jean Baptiste Racine. Sophocles, born at about 496 B.C.E., was friends with the famed historian Herodotus, who traveled extensively throughout Ancient Egypt and wrote extensively on the mysteries (theater) of the Ancient Egyptian Temple.

Masks have a long history of use in African ritual and religious culture. Their use augments the ritual and drama of the myth reenactment and lead the participants to experience a greater intensity of the transcendent and immanent moment. The goal is to get into or become one with the absolute and infinite spirit which abides in all, transcending time. The mask and the process of the religious drama act to assist in leaving the ego consciousness and developing an awareness of the deeper spirit consciousness within.

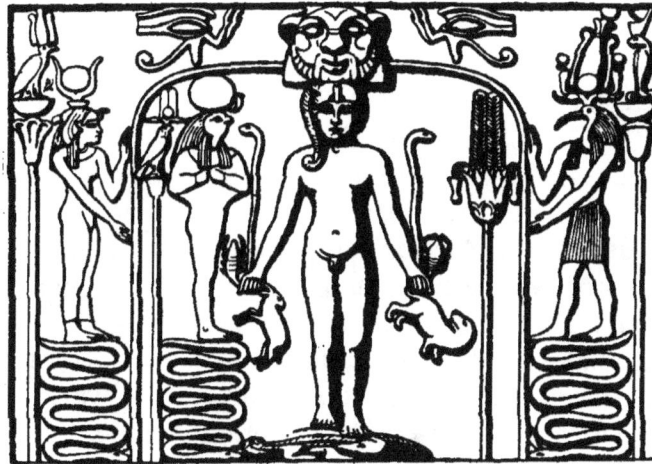

Above -Heru as a Divine child, master of nature, controller of beasts (evil, unrighteousness, the lower self), wearing mask of Basu.

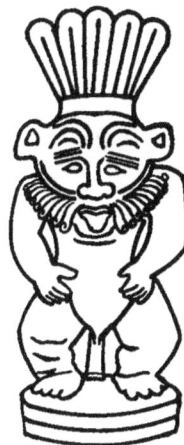

Above right – Basu as the dwarf with the characteristic Nubian plumes as headdress.

The Bas mask he wears is a symbol of the wonderful and magnificent nature of the Divine, who manifests as a dwarf, and at the same time as a personality overflowing with joviality and life.

African religions recognize powers that emanate from the Supreme Being that circulate in the universe like a kind of *life force*. For example, the Dogon worship Amma, the Supreme Being, whose vital force, operates throughout the universe, and is called *Nyama*. The Igbo of southeastern Nigeria call the Supreme Being Chiukwu or Chineke, and the life force that operates in the universe is known as *Chi*. (Which is incidentally also the name for the life force in Chinese and Japanese spirituality.) Another example is to be found in Ancient Egyptian religion with the concept of Neberdjer, the Supreme Being, and Sekhem as the life force which operates throughout the universe. In this manner, the life force itself is to be understood as an intelligent cosmic energy which pervades all of Creation, sustaining it at all times and thereby also unifying it as well.

In African religion the Supreme Being is viewed as a transcendental essence which cannot be defined and therefore cannot be approached directly. One important reason given as to why the lesser spirit powers are invoked while the Supreme Being is seldom invoked or the recipient of offerings is that the Supreme Being, as the ultimate and all-pervasive power in the universe, already owns all and can therefore, receive nothing. For this reason representations of the Supreme Being do not occur in African religions, only the manifesting aspects are given form. These are used to promote the religious movement of the individual by allowing the individual to approach and understand a concrete aspect of the transcendental Spirit. This understanding of course relates to the higher, mystical aspect of religion. Thus, in African religion we see a consistent pattern of structure in the way in which the Spirit is presented across the panorama of African nations. This structure is simple, but extremely profound in conceptualization: The transcendental Supreme Being manifests as lesser or associated powers that emanate from the ultimate source (the same Supreme Being). There are also human beings that, through virtue, become higher powers, i.e. gods and goddesses. Thus, the higher concept behind the practice of ancestor worship in African religion is not of worshipping the souls of the departed relatives, but of propitiating the saints (deified forbears, i.e. canonized) and sages of the past who have elevated themselves and who have become part of the cosmic forces of the Supreme Being. This pattern holds true for African Religions including Ancient Egyptian religion. Again, this is the same course taken by the Western religions, although they do not admit nor profess to view the angels and saints in this way, in practice, many of the followers of those religions worship the angels and saints in the same fashion as within African Religion.

In most African religions, including the Ancient Egyptian, masks, headdress, costumes, the impersonation of lesser divinities are used as means to attract and propitiate the lesser spirits.

African Masks

African masks are an integral part of African culture, art and spirituality. The mask tradition came to its height in Benin and Kamit. The following are examples of the Mask Art as it is used to related the earth realm to the spiritual realm through ritual.

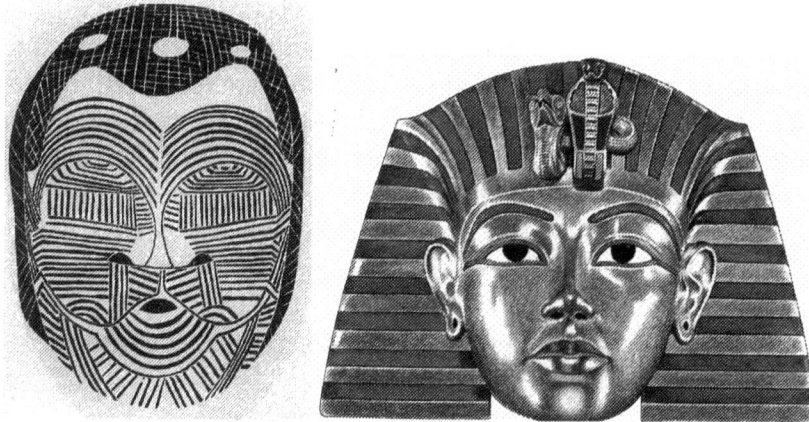

Above left: Typical African Ritual Mask (Congo-Kinshasa) . Right Death of King Tutankhamun of Kamit

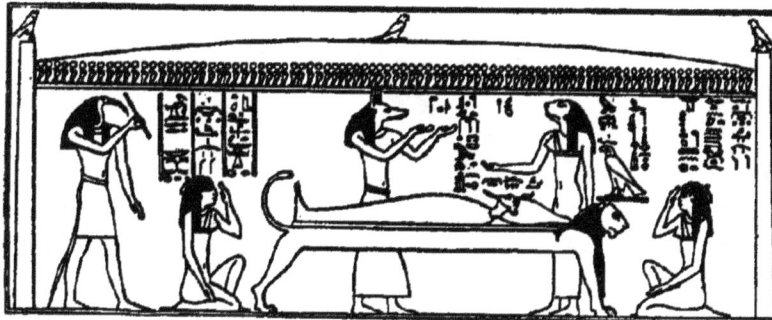

Above: Ancient Egyptian priest performs the rites of the dead while wearing a mask in the likeness of the god Anpu, the divinity of embalming.

Greek Philosophy and Ancient Egyptian Philosophy

The term 'Hellenism' refers to the culture of classical Greece. It is most particularly associated with Athens during the 5th century B.C.E. Thucydides and Herodotus exemplified the writing of history, and Socrates (469-399 B.C.E.), followed by Plato (427-347 B.C.E.), his disciple, established standards for philosophy. Although Euripides did not identify himself with any specific school of philosophy, he was influenced by such philosophers as Socrates.

Socrates (470?-399? B.C.E.) was regarded as one of the most important philosophers of ancient Greece. He ended up spending most of his life in Athens, however, he was known to have studied under the Ionian philosophers. The Ionian school of Greek philosophy was founded by Thales (600 B.C.E.?) who was a direct student of the Ancient Egyptian sages. This establishes a direct link between Socrates and his teachings with Ancient Egypt. Socrates had a tremendous influence on many disciples. One of the most popular of these was Plato. Plato in turn taught others including Aristotle (384-322 B.C.E.), who was Plato's disciple for 19 years. After Plato's death, Aristotle opened a school of philosophy in Asia Minor. Aristotle educated Philip of Macedon's son, Alexander (Alexander the Great), between the years 343 and 334 B.C.E., and then returned to Athens and opened a school in the Lyceum (the school near Athens where Aristotle lectured to his students). He urged Alexander on to his conquests since in the process, he, Aristotle, was able to gain in knowledge from the ancient writings of the conquered countries. After Alexander's conquest of Egypt, Aristotle is said to have become the author of over 1,000 books on philosophy. Building on Plato's theory of the Forms, Aristotle developed the theory of the *Unmoved Mover* which is a direct teaching from Memphite Theology of Ancient Egypt. Among his works are De Anima, Nicomachean Ethics and Metaphysics.

Tracing the Influence of Ancient Egyptian Theater:

Ancient Egyptian Theater
⬇
Greek Theater
⬇
Roman Theater
⬇
Christian Theater
⬇
Modern Western Theater

Many people believe that the art of theater began with the ancient Greek theater. Thespis, the first actor-dramatist (about 560 B.C.E.), is considered to have been the first person to give the Greek drama its form; actors are still called "thespians." However, upon closer examination, it must be noted that just as Greek philosophers such as Thales and Pythagoras learned their wisdom from the Ancient Egyptians and then set up their schools of philosophy in Greece, it is likely that the first Greek actors and playwrights learned their profession from the Ancient Egyptian Sages when they came from Greece to learn the religion and the sciences. (see the book "From Egypt to Greece" by Muata Ashby available through the Sema Institute and bookstores.) Actually, a great debt is owed to the Greek writers of ancient times because their records attest to many details which the Ancient Egyptians did not record.

There was no public theater in Ancient Egypt as the modern world knows theater at present. Theater in present day society is performed publicly for the main purpose of entertainment, but in Ancient Egypt the theatrical performances were reserved for the temple exclusively. This was because the performing arts, including music, were held to be powerful and sacred endeavors which were used to impart spiritual teachings and evoke spiritual feeling, and were not to be used as frivolous forms of entertainment. The Greek writer, Strabo, relates that multitudes of people would flock to festival centers (important cities and temples) where the scenes from myths about the gods and goddesses would be acted out.

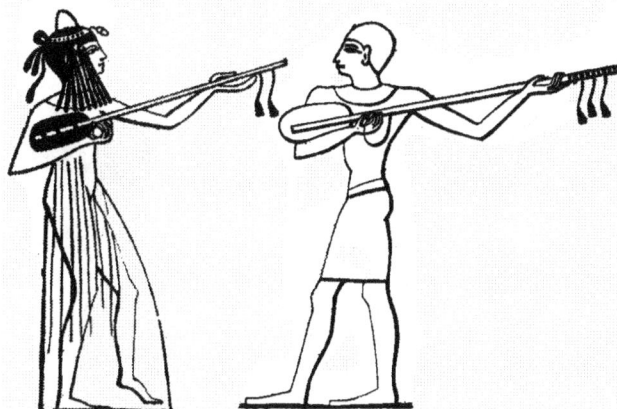

Ancient Egyptian Lute Players

Sometimes the main episodes of the religious dramas were performed outside the temple, in the courtyard or between the pylons, of the "Paristyle Hall" or "Hypostyle Hall" areas and were the most important attraction of the festivals. The most esoteric (mystical) elements were performed in the interior portion of the temple for initiates, priests and priestesses only. (see the temple diagram- Images From the Temple of Hetheru) The priests and priestesses took great care with costumes and the decorations (direction and set design). The spectators knew the myths that were being acted out but never stopped enjoying their annual performance, being a retelling of the divine stories, which bring purpose and meaning to life. Thus, the art of acting was set aside for spiritual purposes and was not to be used for mindless entertainment, which serves only to distract the mind from reality and truth. The spectators would take part by clapping, lamenting at sad parts, crying out with joy and celebrating when the ultimate triumph came. In this manner the spectators became part of the myth. As the myth is essentially about the life of the gods and goddesses, and it is their lives that not only sustain the world, but also leads to understanding the connection between the physical, material and spiritual worlds, the reenactment of these dramas serve to teach and reinforce in the general population, the spiritual values of the Kamitan (Kemetic) culture. Further, the occasions were used as opportunities for enjoying life, though it was understood to be fleeting. Thus, the bridge between the mortal world and the eternal world was established, through mythological drama and the performing arts.

In the Ancient Egyptian view, life cannot be enjoyed without affirming the Divine, the Spirit. Further, theater, religion and mystical philosophy were considered to be aspects of the same discipline, known as "Shetaut Neter" or the "mysteries" or "Yoga Sciences." Every aspect of life in Ancient Egypt was permeated by the awareness and inclusion of spiritual philosophy. For example, lawyers and judges followed the precepts of Maat, and medical doctors followed and worshipped the teachings of the god Djehuti, who was adopted by the Greeks as the god Asclapius. This idea is also evident in the Ancient Egyptian manner of saying grace before meals even by ordinary householders. Prior to consuming food, the host of an ordinary household would invite the guests to view an image of a divinity, principally Asar (Osiris) the god of the afterlife, thereby reminding the guests that life is fleeting, even as they are about to enjoy a sumptuous meal. In this manner, a person is reminded of the ultimate fate and purpose of life and a reflective state of mind is engendered rather than an arrogant and egoistic state. This theme is present in every aspect of Ancient Egyptian culture at its height.

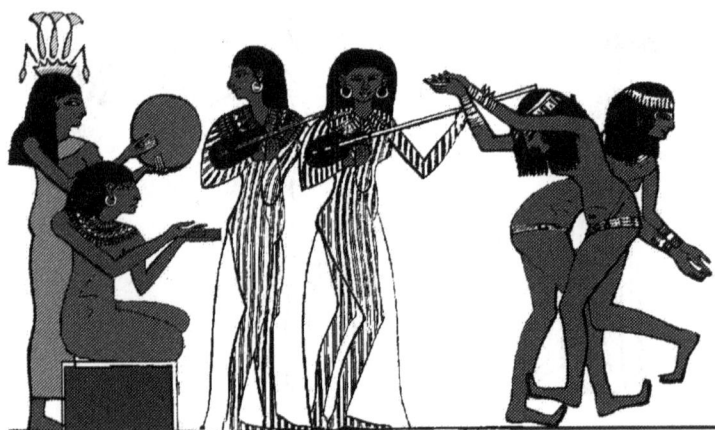

Ancient Egyptian female musicians playing the Lute and Hand Drum while two others dance.

The Ancient Egyptian Sages instituted tight controls on theater and music because the indulgence in inappropriate entertainments was known to cause mental agitation and undesirable behaviors. The famous Greek Philosopher and student of the Ancient Egyptian Mysteries, Pythagoras, wrote that the Ancient Egyptians placed particular attention to the study of music. Another famous Greek Philosopher and student of the Ancient Egyptian Mysteries, Plato, states that they thought it was beneficial to the youths. Strabo confirms that music was taught to youths along with reading and writing, however, it was understood that music meant for entertainment alone was harmful to the mind, making it agitated and difficult to control oneself, and thus was strictly controlled by the state and the priests and priestesses. Like the sages of India, who instituted Nada Yoga, or the spiritual path of music, the Ancient Egyptians held that music was of Divine origin and as such was a sacred endeavor. The Greek writer, Athenaeus, informs us that the Greeks and barbarians from other countries learned music from the Ancient Egyptians. Music was so important in Ancient Egypt that professional musicians were contracted and kept on salaries at the temples. Music was considered important because it has the special power to carry the mind to either elevated (spiritual) states or (worldly) states. When there is overindulgence in music for entertainment and escapism (tendency to desire to escape from daily routine or reality by indulging in fantasy, daydreaming, or entertainment) or to promote other egoistic experiences (violence, hate, lust, greed, sentimentality, desire, etc.) the mind becomes filled with worldly impressions, cravings, lusting, and uncontrolled urges. In this state of mind, the capacity for right thinking and feeling are distorted or incapacitated. The advent of audio and visual recording technology and their combinations in movies and music videos, is more powerful because the visual element, coupled with music, and the ability to repeat with intensity of volume, acts to intoxicate the mind with illusory, egoistic and fantasy thoughts. The body is also affected in this process. The vibrations of the music and the feelings contained in it through the lyrics and sentiment of the performer evokes the production of certain psychological and corresponding bio-chemical processes in the mind and body, respectively. This capacity of music is evident in movies musicals, converts, audio recordings, etc., in their capacity to change a person's mood. Any and all messages given to the mind affect it, and therefore, great care should be taken to fill the mind with the right kinds of messages in the form of sublime ideas and feelings.

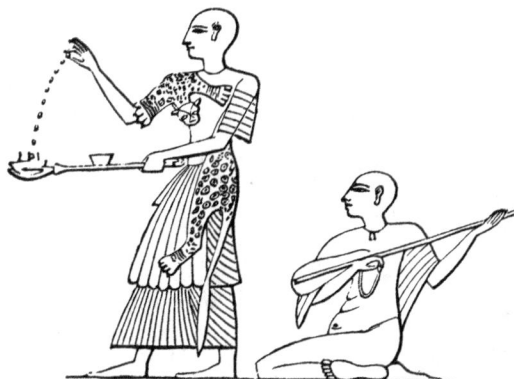

Ancient Egyptian priests – one playing the Lute and the other burns incense

Those societies which produce and consume large quantities of audio and audio-visual entertainment for non-spiritual purposes will exhibit the greatest levels of cultural degradation which will express as mental agitation, violence, individual frustration, addiction, mental illness, physical illness, etc., no matter how materially prosperous or technologically advanced they may become. So true civilization and success of a society should not be judged by material prosperity or technological advancement, but rather by how successful it is in producing the inner fulfillment of its citizens. Being the creators of and foremost practitioners of Maat Philosophy (adherence to the principles of righteousness in all aspects of life- See the book "The Wisdom of Maati" by Dr. Muata Ashby), the Ancient Egyptians created a culture which existed longer (at least 5,000 years) than any other known society and the construction methods of many of their monuments still defy explanation and cannot be duplicated. Therefore, the real measures of civilization and human evolution are to be discerned by the emphasis on and refinement of the performing and visual arts and spiritual philosophy, for these endeavors serve to bring harmony to the individual and to society. (The word spiritual here implies any endeavor which seeks to bring understanding about the ultimate questions of life: Who am I? and What is life all about? So spirituality may or may not be related to organized religion.) It should be clearly understood that art should not become stagnant or rigid in its expression since this is the means by which it is renewed for the understanding of new generations. Rather, the principles contained in the arts should be kept intact in the performance of the rituals, paintings, sculptures, music, etc., since these reflect transcendental truths which are as effective today as they were 5,000 years ago in the Ancient Egyptian temple and will be effective until the end of time. The loss of these is the cause of disharmony in society, but societal dysfunction is in reality only a reflection of disharmony in the individual human heart which has lost its connection with the Higher Self within.

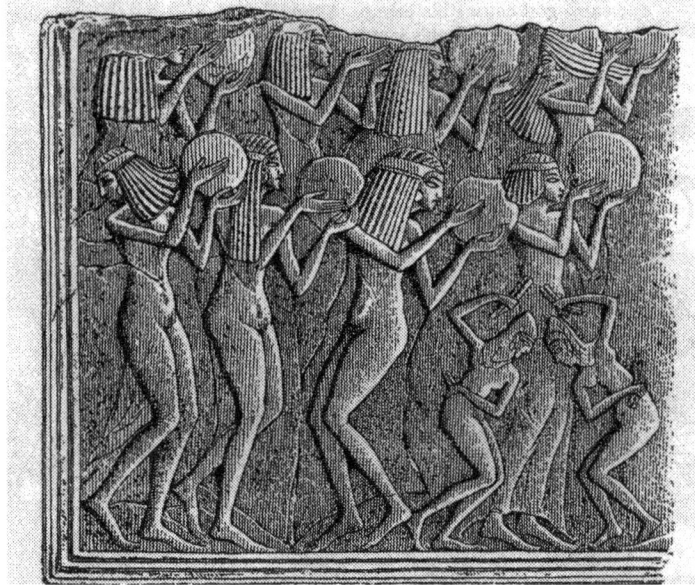

Ancient Egyptian female dancers playing the hand drums and clappers (Two flat pieces of wood held between the fingers and struck together rhythmically.)

Dance and certain special physical movements were also an important part of Ancient Egyptian life. Dance, along with music, was used to worship the gods and goddesses, especially Asar and Hetheru.

Certain special physical postures that may be referred to as *Tjef Neteru Sema Paut* or *Movements of the Gods and Goddesses* were practiced by the priests and priestesses. They are a form of ritualized emulation of the divinities. The original depictions can be seen on temple walls as well as papyrus inscriptions. The main images of Sema Paut can be seen below. For more information see the book *Egyptian Yoga Movements of the Gods and Goddesses* by Muata Ashby.

Figure 1: The varied postures found in the Kamitan papyruses and temple inscriptions.

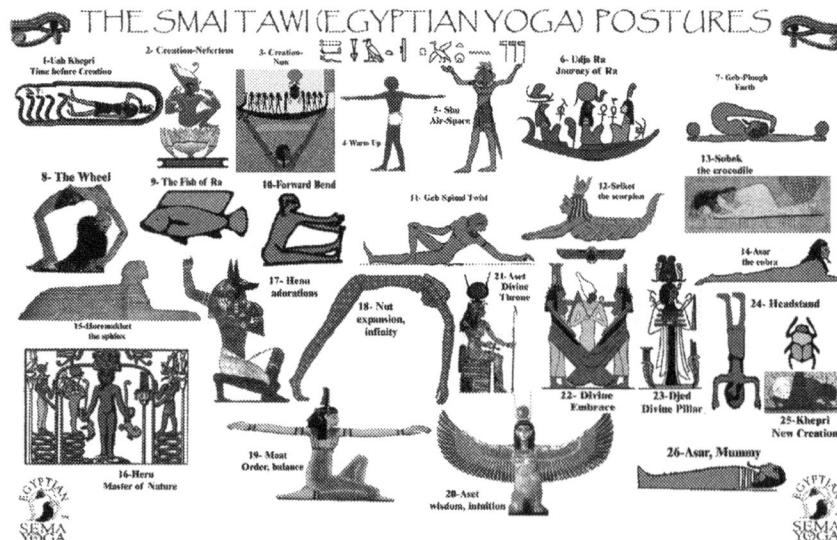

Figure 2: The practice of the postures is shown in the sequence below.

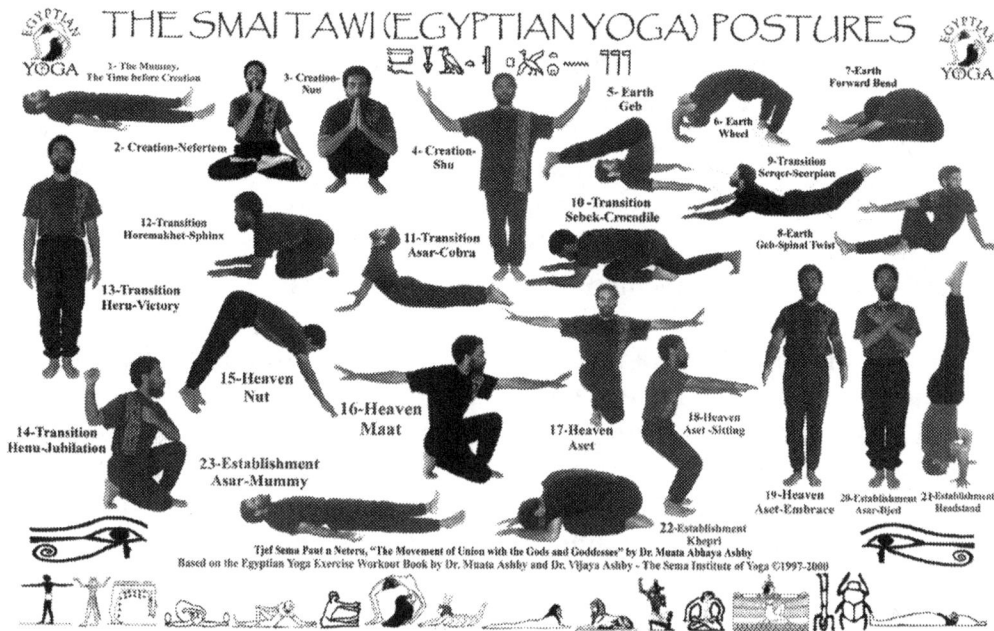

One important dramatic reenactment was the battle of Heru and Set, the two rivals for the throne of Ancient Egypt. Set represents the forces of deceit and unrighteousness. Heru represents the forces of righteousness and order.

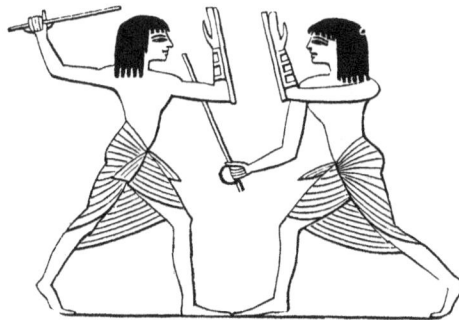

The two contenders

However, dance was also present in private dinner parties. Also, private parties were the scene for entertainments such as games (such as Senet-similar to modern day Parcheesi), juggling, mimes, music and limited theatrical performances. Men and women would dance together or alone and would improvise more than in the dances of the temples and special ceremonies. As is the custom in modern day India and Japan, the Ancient Egyptians would take off their shoes when entering a house or the temple as a sign of reverence for the host and a symbolic gesture of leaving the world outside when practicing higher endeavors.

Thus, the question of whether or not music and entertainment has an effect on youth and the mind of a person was resolved in ancient times. The Ancient Egyptians observed that the people from Greece and the Asiatic countries were more aggressive, and that their behavior was unstable. (See the books Egyptian Yoga Vol. 1 and 2 and The 42 Laws of Maat and the Wisdom Texts) They attributed these problems to their lifestyle, which was full of strife due to life in harsh geographical regions, meat eating and overindulgence in sense pleasures, and the inability to control the human urges and the consequent disconnection from the natural order of the universe as well as the spiritual inner self. These observations of the psychology and lifestyle of the foreigners prompted the Ancient Egyptian Sages to refer to the Greeks and Asiatics (Middle Easterners) as "children" and "miserable"..."barbarians." Their observations allowed the Ancient Egyptian Sages to create a philosophy of life and a psycho-spiritual environment wherein the Kamitic people could grow and thrive in physical, mental and spiritual health.

In ancient Greece, theater became a practice which was open to the public, and later on in the Christian era it deteriorated into mindless entertainment or a corrupted endeavor of con artists. In present times it is a big business, a show business, wherein its participants are paid excessive and disproportionately high salaries for their entertainment skills; or otherwise said, their ability to sell merchandise. In modern times the almost unfettered creation and promotion of movies, videos, music and other forms of entertainment containing elements designed to promote sense pleasures and excitement, leads to mental agitation, but with little true satisfaction of the inner need of the heart. Thus, while the entertainments may cause excitation, they do not lead to abiding fulfillment and inner peace, but to more desires for more excitement in a never ending cycle which is impossible to fulfill. This process leads to mental confusion and stress which in turn lead to strife and conflict, internal frustration. Corresponding with the emergence of Western and Middle Eastern culture, with its negative lifestyle elements noted by the Ancient Egyptians, the world has also seen an increase in wars, violence against women, children, environmental destruction, enslavement and taking advantage of weaker human beings, drug abuse, crime, divorce, and overall personal dissatisfaction with life. In other words, the lack of restraints, in both individuals and in societies as a whole, has led to frustration with life, a kind of cultural depression and degradation, which has led to record numbers of people suffering from mental illnesses such as depression, schizophrenia, psychosis, as well as medical disorders of all kinds which were not present in ancient times due to self-control and the direction of life being guided by spiritual pursuits as opposed to egoistic pursuits. The Ancient Egyptian Mystery theater provides the means for allowing a human being to come into harmony with the spiritual reality (mental expansion and self-discovery) while frivolous entertainment serves to dull the intellectual capacity to discover and understand anything beyond the physical world and the physical sense pleasures of life (mental contraction and hardening of the ego). This inability to go beyond sense pleasures and experiences the world of human activity is what leads a person to mental stress, which in turn leads to mental illness and physical illness.

Therefore, understanding the message of Ancient Egyptian Theater is of paramount importance to human evolution. In Ancient Egypt, theater and music were used for spiritual education and to maintain harmony between the individual and the universe, the soul and the Divine. Thus, spiritual plays were acted by the priests and priestesses, initiates and sometimes by the relatives of the deceased (especially in the case of the Pert Em Heru Mysteries). The use of masks in theater did not originate in Greece. Their use already existed in Ancient Egypt. Unlike the Greek theater, which placed great importance on tragedy in life, masks, such as those presented in this volume were sometimes used by those playing the characters of the mystery in an effort to understand the mystery by becoming one with it, to embody the qualities of the divinity being portrayed and in so doing ultimately becoming one with the Divine. Also, the purpose was to promote the well being of others by directing one's mind and heart towards what is righteous, beautiful and good in the world and beyond. This was the motivation and source of strength which allowed Ancient Egyptian Culture, led by the priests and priestesses, to achieve a high degree of "civilization" and spiritual enlightenment.

Thus the earliest religious rituals in Egypt were performed as plays which were often part of festival periods. This tradition began with the early dynastic period and the Asarian Resurrection myth (5,000 B.C.E. or earlier), which surrounds the death and resurrection of the god Asar (Osiris). This was the main play that was performed universally in Kamit and then in Greece and Rome in later times after the Greeks came to Kamit to learn the arts, sciences, and spiritual philosophy upon which then established their civilization. In Ancient Egypt the story of Hetheru was revered so highly that an annual play and festivity was held in her honor which commemorated her saga, even down to the early Christian era. It was so popular that it was observed widely throughout the entire country of Egypt. Remnants of it and other Ancient Egyptian festivals, survive even today in the rituals of the Muslims who live in present day Egypt. Thus, theater emerged in ancient Africa and influenced Europe, and what would later develop into Greek and Christian theater. The practice of the mystery play was done for the purpose of worshipping the goddess, and also as a method of imparting some important mystical teachings. These have been presented at length in the gloss following the presentation of the play, which discusses the main themes of the myth of Hetheru. Therefore, anyone wishing to learn more about the teachings and practice of Ancient Egyptian philosophy can learn much from participating in the play and studying Ancient Egyptian Philosophy (Shetaut Neter-Smai Tawi-Ancient Egyptian or Kamitic Yoga).

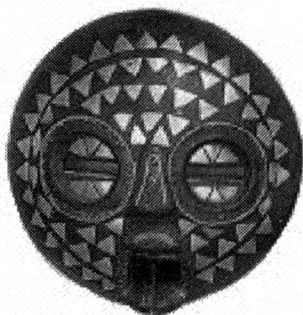 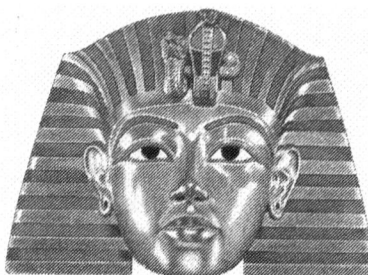 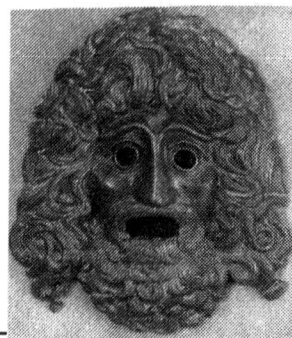

A- Baluba mask of Ghana, B- Mask of Tutankhamun, C- Ancient Greek tragedy mask

Reenactment of the Mysteries

Below: Lord Anpu priest embalming the god Asar as goddess Aset and goddess Nebthet look on. One of the common reenactments is of the mummification and resurrection of Asar.

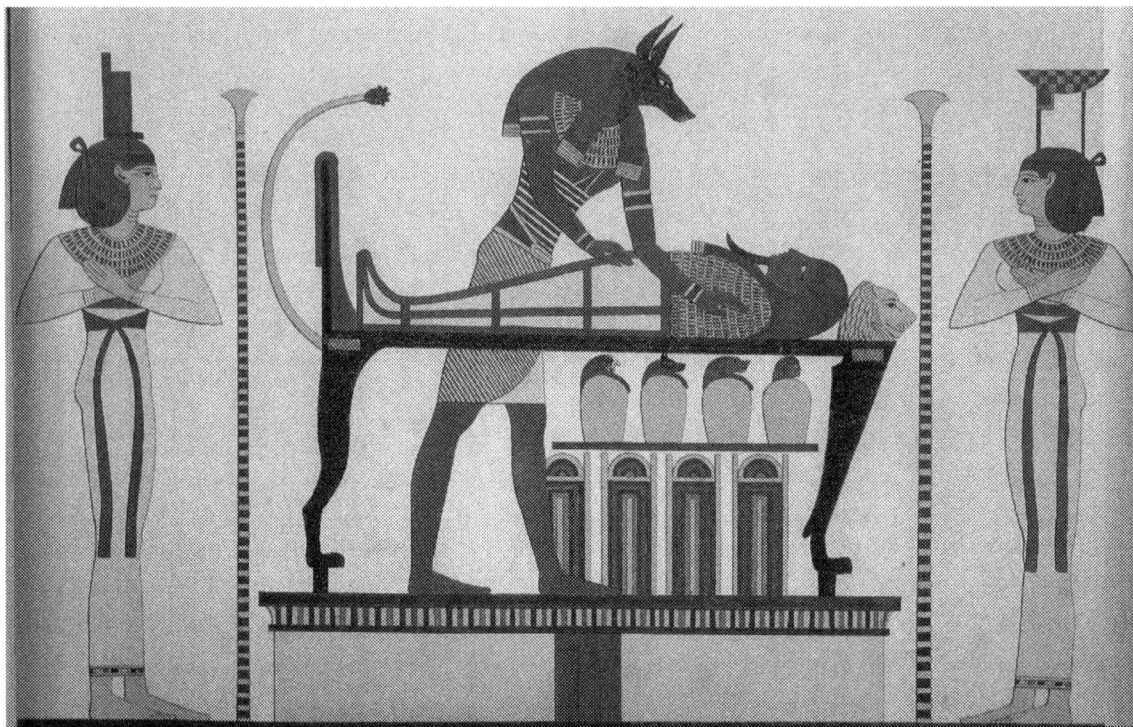

One of the main duties of the advanced priesthood (not the lower ranks) is the reenactment of the myths of the tutelary Divinity of the Temple. This reenactment is the ritual in the form of a theatrical performance and has the effect of promoting a communal meditative experience in the participants in which they eventually identify with the Divinity whose drama is being reenacted.

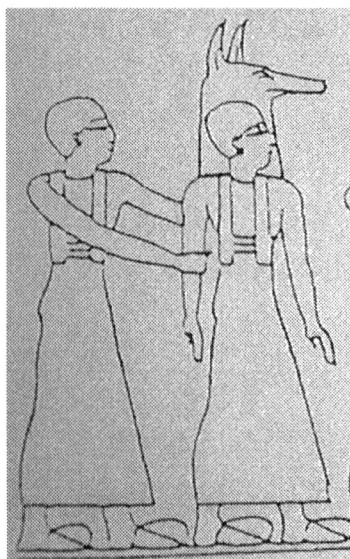

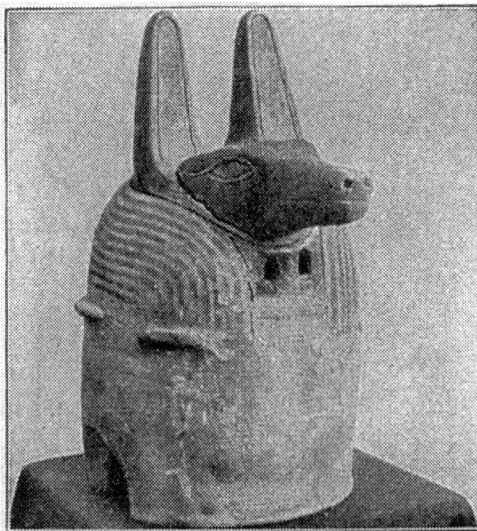

At left: Actually, the character of Anpu is an Ancient Egyptian priest who performs the rites of the dead while wearing a mask/helmet having the likeness of the god Anpu (actual surviving Anpu helmet - above right), who is the divinity of embalming.

Below: The priest as Anpu holds the mummy of Asar Ani upright.

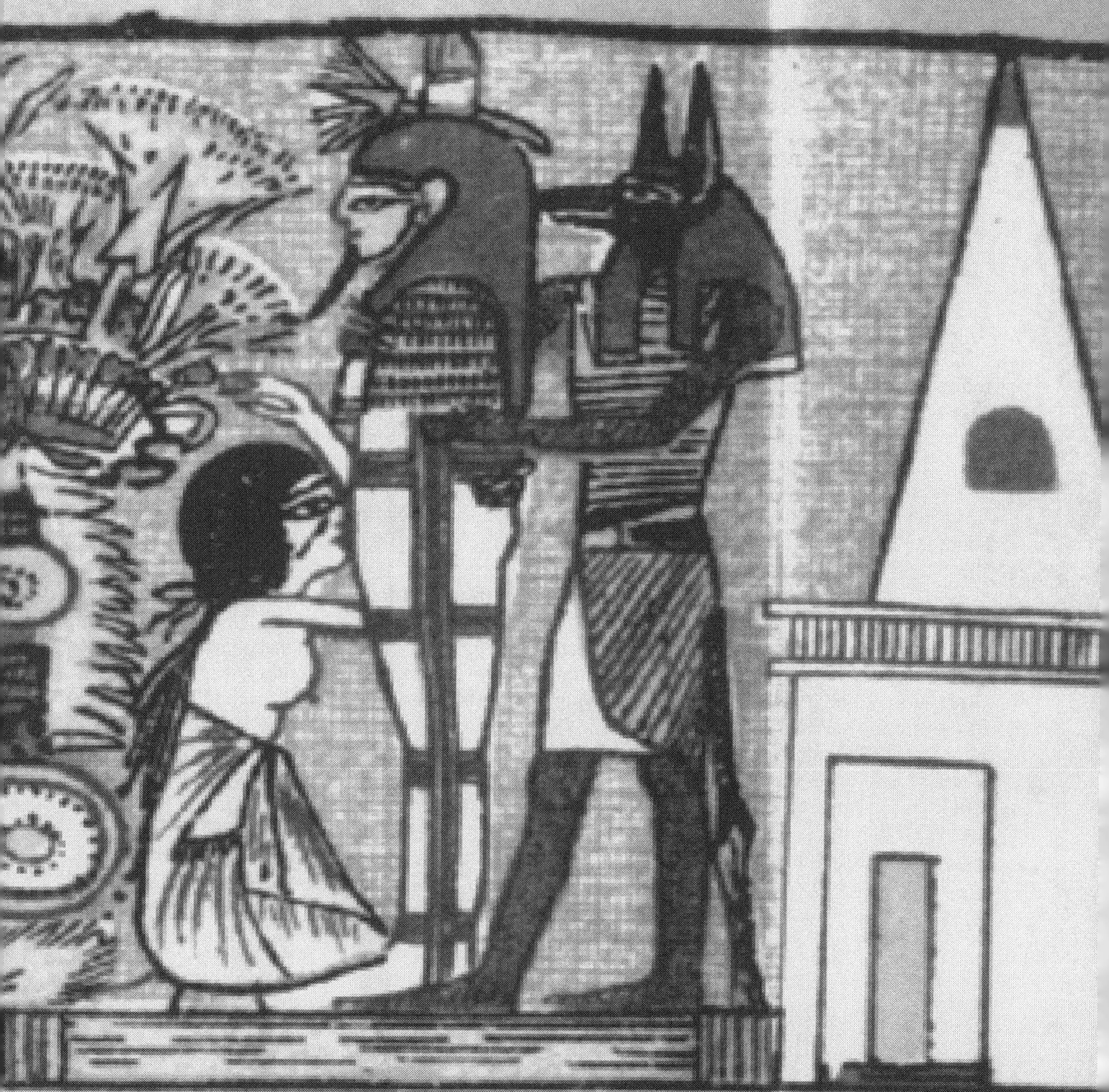

THE RELIGION OF ANCIENT EGYPT

The work of the ancient Egyptian temple is essentially the reenactment of the Neterian Myths and the recreation of the actions of the gods and goddesses based on the religious teaching and philosophy of the ancient Egyptian gods and goddesses, developed by the priests and priestesses. A full treatment of Ancient Egyptian religion is impossible in this small booklet. However, there are some important factors to understand about Ancient Egyptian religion and Yoga Philosophy. The first sophisticated system of religion and yoga mystical philosophy in historical times (5,000 B.C.E.) occurred in Ancient Egypt. This system included all of the gods and goddesses which in later times became individually popular in various cities throughout Ancient Egypt. At the heart of this system of gods and goddesses was *Shetai*, the hidden and unmanifest essence of the universe, also known as *Neberdjer* and *Amun*. The system of religion of Ancient Egypt was called *Shetaut Neter* or the *Hidden Way of The Unmanifest Supreme Being*.

The entire system of mystical philosophy of the hidden Supreme Being, as well as the method through which that Being manifests in the form of the phenomenal physical universe and individual human consciousness, was explained in progressive stages in the theology of the Trinity known as Amun-Ra-Ptah, which was said to have arisen out of the Supreme Being: Neberdjer. As Ancient Egyptian history moved on through thousands of years, each segment of this Trinity was adopted by a particular priesthood and locality which then set about to explain and expound the philosophy of that particular segment of the Trinity. The priests of the Ancient Egyptian city of Anu adopted Ra, the priesthood of the Ancient Egyptian city of Hetkaptah adopted Ptah, and the Ancient Egyptian city of Waset or Newt (Thebes) adopted Amun.[9]

Fundamental Concepts of Kamitan Spirituality

Ancient Egyptian Religion is predicated upon a simple but profound concept which is based in the mystical experience. Elevated initiates discovered that all Creation is actually an expression of one indivisible being. That being manifests as the apparent objects and multiplicity in Creation. This being was referred to as "Neter" and its expressions were termed "Neteru." Neter means "Divinity" and Neteru means "Aspects of the original divinity." Another term that is used to describe the neteru is "Gods and Goddesses." The gods and goddesses are like the children and the Supreme Being, Neter, is the ultimate parent of all. This Ancient Egyptian system of divinities was adopted by the Ancient Greeks by their own admission. Therefore, it is no surprise to see that the fundamental concepts, iconographies and many aspects of Greek mythology appear to be copies of the earlier Ancient Egyptian creations. This religion centers around the concept of the single, undivided being. Therefore, the religion of Ancient Egypt may be referred to as "Neterianism." The following is an overview of Ancient Egyptian religious philosophy.

---

[9] See *Egyptian Yoga Vol. I: The Philosophy of Enlightenment* and *Egyptian Yoga Vol. II: The Supreme Wisdom of Enlightenment* by Dr. Muata Ashby

The Fundamental Principles of Ancient Egyptian Religion

NETERIANISM
(The Oldest Known Religion in History)

The term "Neterianism" is derived from the name "Shetaut Neter." Shetaut Neter means the "Hidden Divinity." It is the ancient philosophy and mythic spiritual culture that gave rise to the Ancient Egyptian civilization. Those who follow the spiritual path of Shetaut Neter are therefore referred to as "Neterians." The fundamental principles common to all denominations of Ancient Egyptian Religion may be summed up in four "Great Truths" that are common to all the traditions of Ancient Egyptian Religion.

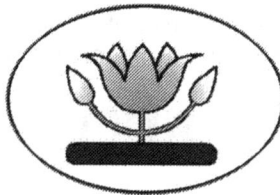

Summary of Ancient Egyptian Religion

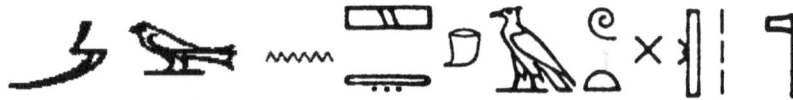

Maa Ur n Shetaut Neter

"Great Truths of The Shetaut Neter Religion"

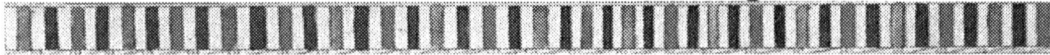

I

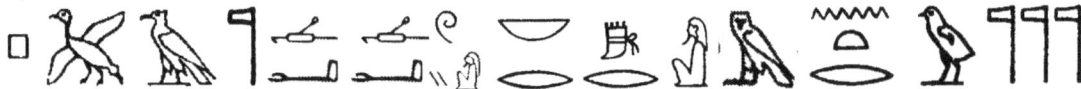

Pa Neter ua ua Neberdjer m Neteru

"The Neter, the Supreme Being, is One and alone and as Neberdjer, manifesting everywhere and in all things in the form of Gods and Goddesses."

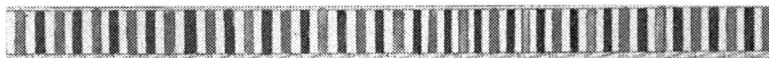

II

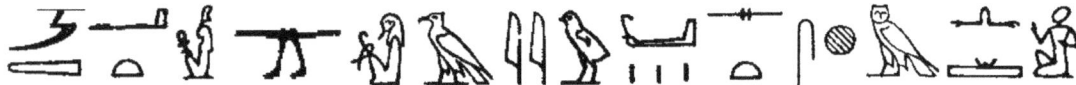

an-Maat swy Saui Set s-Khemn

"Lack of righteousness brings fetters to the personality and these fetters cause ignorance of the Divine."

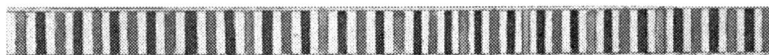

III

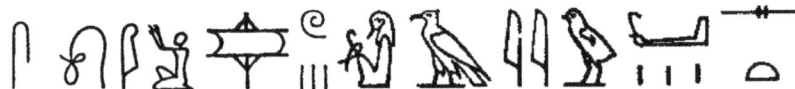

s-Uashu s-Nafu n saiu Set

"Devotion to the Divine leads to freedom from the fetters of Set."

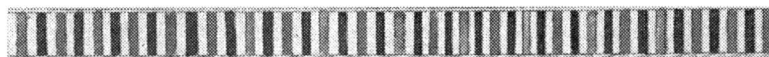

IIII

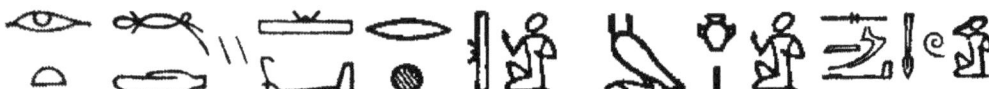

ari Shedy Rekh ab m Maakheru

"The practice of the Shedy disciplines leads to knowing oneself and the Divine. This is called being True of Speech"

Neterian Great Truths

1. ***"Pa Neter ua ua Neberdjer m Neteru"*** -"The Neter, the Supreme Being, is One and alone and as Neberdjer, manifesting everywhere and in all things in the form of Gods and Goddesses."

Neberdjer means "all-encompassing divinity," the all-inclusive, all-embracing Spirit which pervades all and who is the ultimate essence of all. This first truth unifies all the expressions of Kamitan religion.

2. **"an-Maat swy Saui Set s-Khemn"** – "Lack of righteousness brings fetters to the personality and these fetters lead to ignorance of the Divine."

When a human being acts in ways that contradict the natural order of nature, negative qualities of the mind will develop within that person's personality. These are the afflictions of Set. Set is the neteru of egoism and selfishness. The afflictions of Set include: anger, hatred, greed, lust, jealousy, envy, gluttony, dishonesty, hypocrisy, etc. So to be free from the fetters of set one must be free from the afflictions of Set.

3. **"s-Uashu s-Nafu n saiu Set"** -"Devotion to the Divine leads to freedom from the fetters of Set."

To be liberated (Nafu - freedom - to breath) from the afflictions of Set, one must be devoted to the Divine. Being devoted to the Divine means living by Maat. Maat is a way of life that is purifying to the heart and beneficial for society as it promotes virtue and order. Living by Maat means practicing Shedy (spiritual practices and disciplines).

Uashu means devotion and the classic pose of adoring the Divine is called "Dua," standing or sitting with upraised hands facing outwards towards the image of the divinity.

4. **"ari Shedy Rekh ab m Maakheru"** - "The practice of the Shedy disciplines leads to knowing oneself and the Divine. This is called being True of Speech."

Doing Shedy means to study profoundly, to penetrate the mysteries (Shetaut) and discover the nature of the Divine. There have been several practices designed by the sages of Ancient Kamit to facilitate the process of self-knowledge. These are the religious (Shetaut) traditions and the Sema (Smai) Tawi (yogic) disciplines related to them that augment the spiritual practices.

All the traditions relate the teachings of the sages by means of myths related to particular gods or goddesses. It is understood that all of these neteru are related, like brothers and sisters, having all emanated from the same source, the same Supremely Divine parent, who is neither male nor female, but encompasses the totality of the two.

The Great Truths of Neterianism are realized by means of
Four Spiritual Disciplines in Three Steps

The four disciples are: Rekh Shedy (Wisdom), Ari Shedy (Righteous Action and Selfless Service), Uashu (Ushet) Shedy (Devotion) and Uaa Shedy (Meditation)

See the following page

The Three Steps are: Listening, Ritual, and Meditation

SEDJM REKH SHEDY

L I S T E N

- *Sedjm REKH Shedy - Listening to the WISDOM of the Neterian Traditions*

  - Shetaut Asar — Teachings of the Asarian Tradition
  - Shetaut Anu — Teachings of the Ra Tradition
  - Shetaut Menefer — Teachings of the Ptah Tradition
  - Shetaut Waset — Teachings of the Amun Tradition
  - Shetaut Netrit — Teachings of the Goddess Tradition
  - Shetaut Aton — Teachings of the Aton Tradition

ARI SHEDY

R I T U A L

- *Ari Maat Shedy – Righteous Actions – Purifies the GROSS impurities of the Heart*

  - Maat Shedy — True Study of the Ways of hidden nature of Neter
  - Maat Aakhu — True Deeds that lead to glory
  - Maat Aru — True Ritual

UASHU (USHET) SHEDY

- *Ushet Shedy – Devotion to the Divine – Purifies the EMOTIONAL impurities of the Heart*

  - Shmai – Divine Music
  - Sema Paut – Meditation in motion
  - Neter Arit – Divine Offerings – Selfless-Service – virtue -

UAA SHEDY

M E D I T A T E

- *Uaa m Neter Shedy -* 𓏺𓃰𓄿𓏏𓏺 **Meditation** Experience the Transcendental Supreme Self. The five forms of Neterian Meditation discipline include.

  - Arat Sekhem, - Meditation on the Subtle Life Force
  - Ari Sma Maat, - Meditation on the Righteous action
  - Nuk Pu-Ushet, - Meditation on the I am
  - Nuk Ra Akhu, - Meditation on the Glorious Light
  - Rekh – Khemn, -Meditation on the Wisdom Teaching

The Spiritual Culture and the Purpose of Life: Shetaut Neter

"Men and women are to become God-like through a life of virtue
and the cultivation of the spirit through scientific knowledge,
practice and bodily discipline."

-Ancient Egyptian Proverb

The highest forms of Joy, Peace and Contentment are obtained when the meaning of life is discovered. When the human being is in harmony with life, then it is possible to reflect and meditate upon the human condition and realize the limitations of worldly pursuits. When there is peace and harmony in life, a human being can practice any of the varied disciplines designated as Shetaut Neter to promote {his/her} evolution towards the ultimate goal of life, which Spiritual Enlightenment. Spiritual Enlightenment is the awakening of a human being to the awareness of the Transcendental essence which binds the universe and which is eternal and immutable. In this discovery is also the sobering and ecstatic realization that the human being is one with that Transcendental essence. With this realization comes great joy, peace and power to experience the fullness of life and to realize the purpose of life during the time on earth. The lotus is a symbol of Shetaut Neter, meaning the turning towards the light of truth, peace and transcendental harmony.

Shetaut Neter

We have established that the Ancient Egyptians were African peoples who lived in the north-eastern quadrant of the continent of Africa. They were descendants of the Nubians, who had themselves originated from farther south into the heart of Africa at the Great Lakes region, the sources of the Nile River. They created a vast civilization and culture earlier than any other society in known history and organized a nation that was based on the concepts of balance and order as well as spiritual enlightenment. These ancient African people called their land Kamit, and soon after developing a well-ordered society, they began to realize that the world is full of wonders, but also that life is fleeting, and that there must be something more to human existence. They developed spiritual systems that were designed to allow human beings to understand the nature of this secret being who is the essence of all Creation. They called this spiritual system "Shtaut Ntr (Shetaut Neter)."

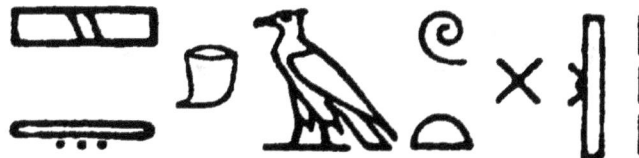

Shetaut means secret.

Neter means Divinity.

Who is Neter in Kamitan Religion?

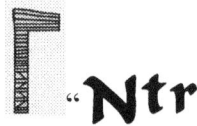

⌐ "**Ntr**

The symbol of Neter was described by an Ancient Kamitan priest as:
"That which is placed in the coffin"

The term Ntr, or Ntjr, comes from the Ancient Egyptian hieroglyphic language which did not record its vowels. However, the term survives in the Coptic language as *"Nutar."* The same Coptic meaning (divine force or sustaining power) applies in the present as it did in ancient times. It is a symbol composed of a wooden staff that was wrapped with strips of fabric, like a mummy. The strips alternate in color with yellow, green and blue. The mummy in Kamitan spirituality is understood to be the dead but resurrected Divinity. So the Nutar (Ntr) is actually every human being who does not really die, but goes to live on in a different form. Further, the resurrected spirit of every human being is that same Divinity. Phonetically, the term Nutar is related to other terms having the same meaning, such as the latin "Natura," the Spanish Naturalesa, the English "Nature" and "Nutriment", etc. In a real sense, as we will see, Natur means power manifesting as Neteru and the Neteru are the objects of creation, i.e. "nature."

Neter and the Neteru

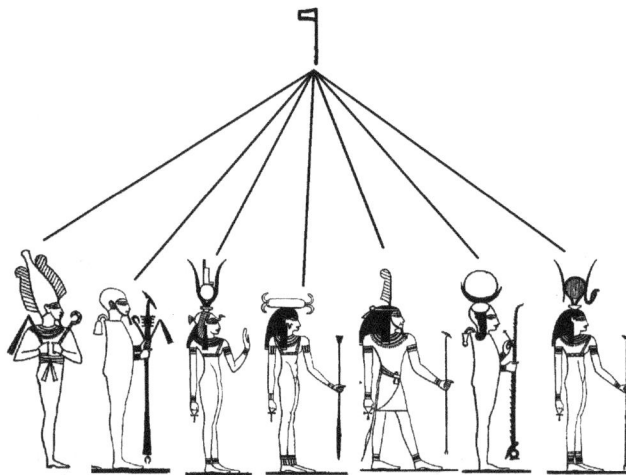

The Neteru (Gods and Goddesses) proceed from the Neter (Supreme Being)

As stated earlier, the concept of Neter and Neteru binds and ties all of the varied forms of Kamitan spirituality into one vision of the gods and goddesses all emerging from the same Supreme Being. Therefore, ultimately, Kamitan spirituality is not polytheistic, nor is it monotheistic, for it holds that the Supreme Being is more than a God or Goddess. The Supreme Being is an all-encompassing Absolute Divinity.

The Neteru

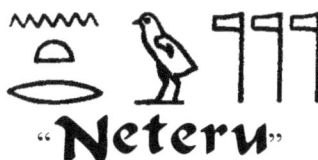

"Neteru"

The term "Neteru" means "gods and goddesses." This means that from the ultimate and transcendental Supreme Being, "Neter," come the Neteru. There are countless Neteru. So from the one come the many. These Neteru are cosmic forces that pervade the universe. They are the means by which Neter sustains Creation and manifests through it. So Neterianism is a monotheistic polytheism. The one Supreme Being expresses as many gods and goddesses. At the end of time, after their work of sustaining Creation is finished, these gods and goddesses are again absorbed back into the Supreme Being.

All of the spiritual systems of Ancient Egypt (Kamit) have one essential aspect that is common to all; they all hold that there is a Supreme Being (Neter) who manifests in a multiplicity of ways through nature, the Neteru. Like sunrays, the Neteru emanate from the Divine; they are its manifestations. So by studying the Neteru we learn about and are led to discover their source, the Neter, and with this discovery we are enlightened. The Neteru may be depicted anthropomorphically or zoomorphically in accordance with the teaching about Neter that is being conveyed through them.

Sacred Scriptures of Shetaut Neter

The following scriptures represent the foundational scriptures of Kamitan culture. They may be divided into three categories: *Mythic Scriptures*, *Mystical Philosophy* and *Ritual Scriptures*, and *Wisdom Scriptures* (Didactic Literature).

MYTHIC SCRIPTURES Literature	Mystical (Ritual) Philosophy Literature	Wisdom Texts Literature
SHETAUT ASAR-ASET-HERU The Myth of Asar, Aset and Heru (Asarian Resurrection Theology) - Predynastic **SHETAUT ATUM-RA** Anunian Theology Predynastic **Shetaut Net/Aset/Hetheru** Saitian Theology – Goddess	**Coffin Texts** (C. 2040 B.C.E.-1786 B.C.E.) **Papyrus Texts** (C. 1580 B.C.E.- Roman Period)[10] Books of Coming Forth By Day	**Wisdom Texts** (C. 3,000 B.C.E. – PTOLEMAIC PERIOD) Precepts of Ptahotep Instructions of Any Instructions of Amenemope Etc. **Maat Declarations** Literature

---

[10] After 1570 B.C.E they would evolve into a more unified text, the Egyptian Book of the Dead.

Spirituality Predynastic **SHETAUT PTAH** Memphite Theology Predynastic Shetaut Amun Theban Theology Predynastic	Example of famous papyri: Papyrus of Any Papyrus of Hunefer Papyrus of Kenna Greenfield Papyrus, Etc.	(All Periods) **Blind Harpers Songs**

The Neteru and Their Temples

Diagram 1: The Ancient Egyptian Temple Network

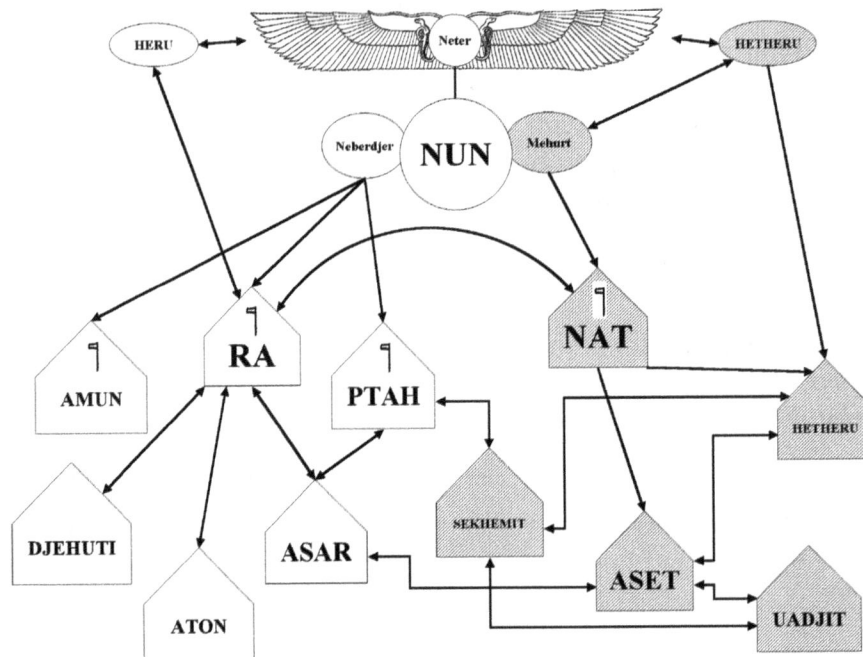

The sages of Kamit instituted a system by which the teachings of spirituality were espoused through a Temple organization. The major divinities were assigned to a particular city. That divinity or group of divinities became the "patron" divinity or divinities of that city. Also, the Priests and Priestesses of that Temple were in charge of seeing to the welfare of the people in that district as well as maintaining the traditions and disciplines of the traditions based on the particular divinity being worshipped. So the original concept of "Neter" became elaborated through the "theologies" of the various traditions. A dynamic expression of the teachings emerged, which though maintaining the integrity of the teachings, expressed nuances of variation in perspective on the teachings to suit the needs of varying kinds of personalities of the people of different locales.

In the diagram above, the primary or main divinities are denoted by the Neter symbol (⌐). The house structure represents the Temple for that particular divinity. The interconnections with the other Temples are based on original scriptural statements espoused by the Temples that linked the divinities of their Temple with the other divinities. So this means that the divinities should be viewed not as separate entities operating independently, but rather as family members who are in the same "business" together, i.e. the enlightenment of society, albeit through variations in form of worship, name, form (expression of the Divinity), etc. Ultimately, all the divinities are referred to as Neteru and they are all said to be emanations from the ultimate and Supreme Being. Thus, the teaching from any of the Temples leads to an understanding of the others, and these all lead back to the source, the highest Divinity. Thus, the teaching within any of the Temple systems would lead to the attainment of spiritual enlightenment, the Great Awakening.

The Neteru and Their Interrelationships

Diagram : The Primary Kamitan Neteru and their Interrelationships

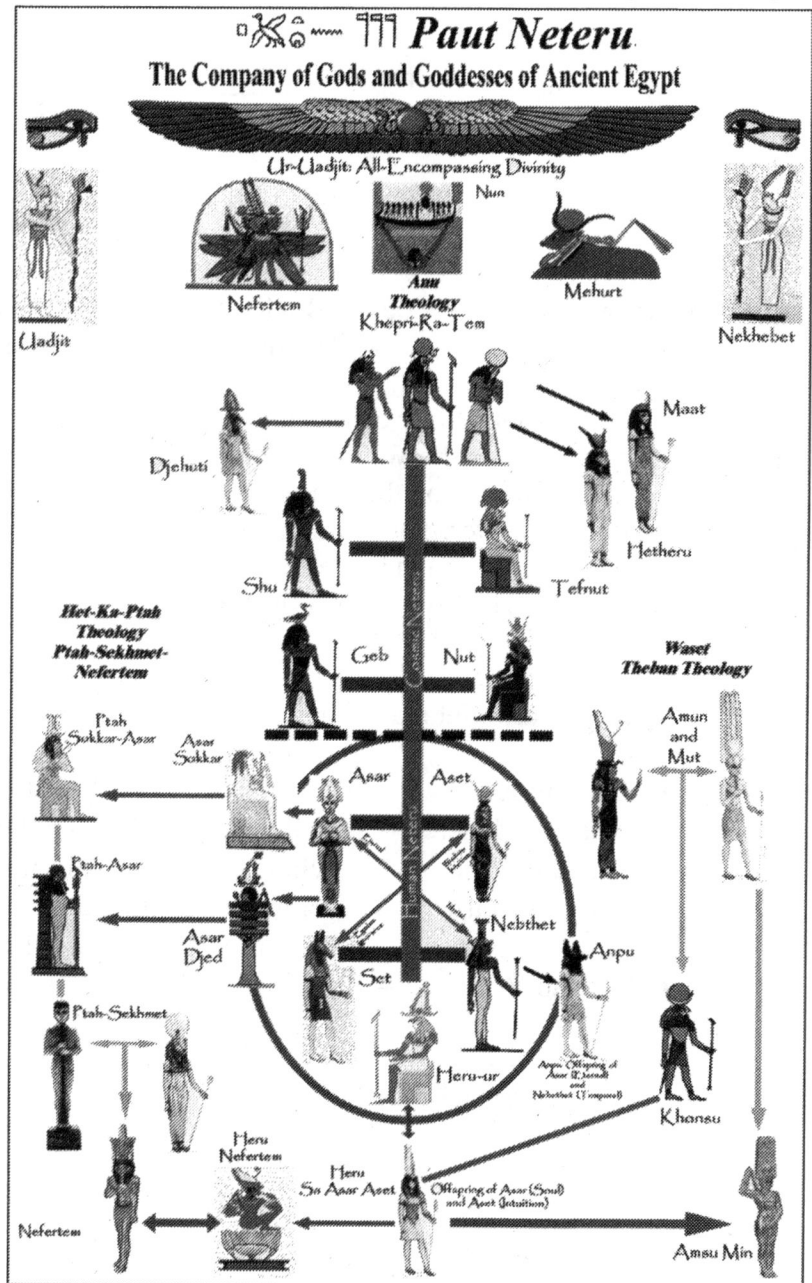

The same Supreme Being, Neter, is the winged all-encompassing transcendental Divinity, the Spirit who, in the early history, is called "Heru." The physical universe in which the Heru lives is called "Hetheru" or the "house of Heru." This divinity (Heru) is also the Nun or primeval substratum from which all matter is composed. The various divinities and the material universe are composed from this primeval substratum. Neter is actually androgynous and Heru, the Spirit, is related as a male aspect of that androgyny. However, Heru in the androgynous aspect, gives rise to the solar principle and this is seen in both the male and female divinities.

The image above provides an idea of the relationships between the divinities of the three main Neterian spiritual systems (traditions): Anunian Theology, Wasetian (Theban) Theology and Het-Ka-Ptah (Memphite) Theology. The traditions are composed of companies or groups of gods and goddesses. Their actions, teachings and interactions with each other and with human beings provide insight into their nature as well as that of human existence and Creation itself. The lines indicate direct scriptural relationships and the labels also indicate that some divinities from one system are the same in others, with only a name change. Again, this is attested to by the scriptures themselves in direct statements, like those found in the *Prt m Hru* text Chapter 4 (17).[11]

Listening to the Teachings

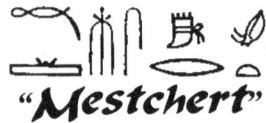

"Mestchert"

"Listening, to fill the ears, listen attentively-"

What should the ears be filled with? The Myths of Shetaut Neter contained in the Traditions of Shetaut Neter

The sages of Shetaut Neter enjoined that a Shemsu Neter (follower of Neter, an initiate or aspirant) should listen to the WISDOM of the Neterian Traditions through special myths. Special rituals were created based on those myths that constitute the basis of the performances of the Ancient Egyptian Theater. These are the myth related to the gods and goddesses containing the basic understanding of who they are, what they represent, how they relate human beings and to the Supreme Being. The myths allow us to be connected to the Divine.

An aspirant may choose any one of the 5 main Neterian Traditions.

- Shetaut Anu   – Teachings of the Ra Tradition
- Shetaut Menefer – Teachings of the Ptah Tradition
- Shetaut Waset   – Teachings of the Amun Tradition
- Shetaut Netrit   – Teachings of the Goddess Tradition
- Shetaut Asar   – Teachings of the Asarian Tradition
- Shetaut Aton   – Teachings of the Aton Tradition

---

[11] See the book *The Egyptian Book of the Dead* by Muata Ashby

The Anunian Tradition

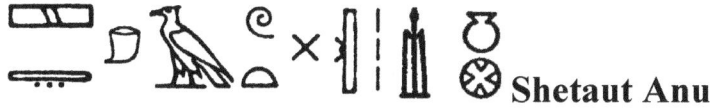

 Shetaut Anu

The Mystery Teachings of the Anunian Tradition are related to the Divinity Ra and his company of Gods and Goddesses.[12] This Temple and its related Temples espouse the teachings of Creation, human origins and the path to spiritual enlightenment by means of the Supreme Being in the form of the god Ra. It tells of how Ra emerged from a primeval ocean and how human beings were created from his tears. The gods and goddesses, who are his children, go to form the elements of nature and the cosmic forces that maintain nature.

Below: The Heliopolitan Cosmogony.

The city of Anu (Amun-Ra)

The Neters of Creation -
The Company of the Gods and Goddesses.
Neter Neteru
Nebertcher - Amun (unseen, hidden, ever present, Supreme Being, beyond duality and description)

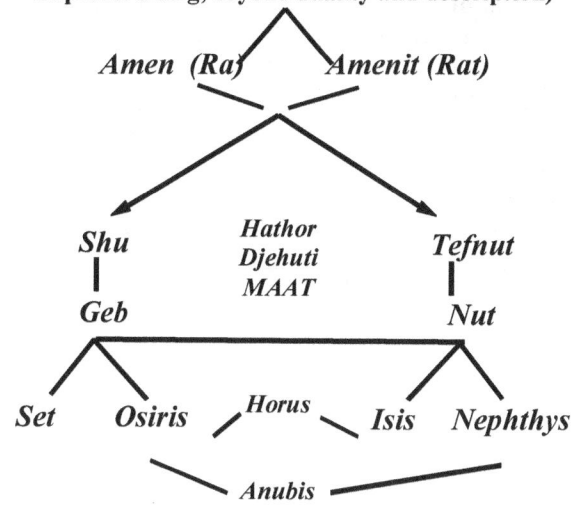

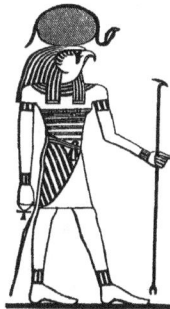

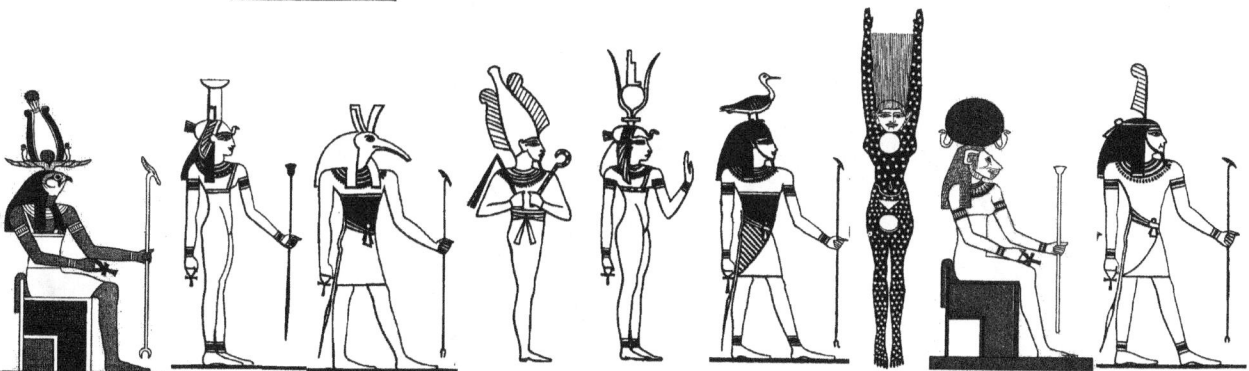

Amen (Ra)   *Amenit (Rat)*

Shu   Hathor   *Tefnut*
          Djehuti
Geb   MAAT   *Nut*

Set *Osiris* *Horus* *Isis* *Nephthys*

Anubis

Top: Ra. From left to right, starting at the bottom level- The Gods and Goddesses of Anunian Theology: Shu, Tefnut, Nut, Geb, Aset, Asar, Set, Nebthet and Heru-Ur

---

[12] See the Book Anunian Theology by Muata Ashby

The Memphite Tradition

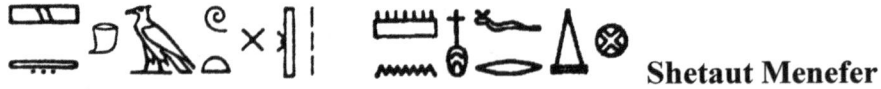

 Shetaut Menefer

The Mystery Teachings of the Menefer (Memphite) Tradition are related to the Neterus known as Ptah, Sekhmit, Nefertem. The myths and philosophy of these divinities constitutes Memphite Theology.[13] This temple and its related temples espoused the teachings of Creation, human origins and the path to spiritual enlightenment by means of the Supreme Being in the form of the god Ptah and his family, who compose the Memphite Trinity. It tells of how Ptah emerged from a primeval ocean and how he created the universe by his will and the power of thought (mind). The gods and goddesses who are his thoughts, go to form the elements of nature and the cosmic forces that maintain nature. His spouse, Sekhmit has a powerful temple system of her own that is related to the Memphite teaching. The same is true for his son Nefertem.

Below: The Memphite Cosmogony.

The city of Hetkaptah (Ptah)

The Neters of Creation -
The Company of the Gods and Goddesses.
Neter Neteru
Nebertcher - Amun (unseen, hidden, ever present, Supreme Being, beyond duality and description)

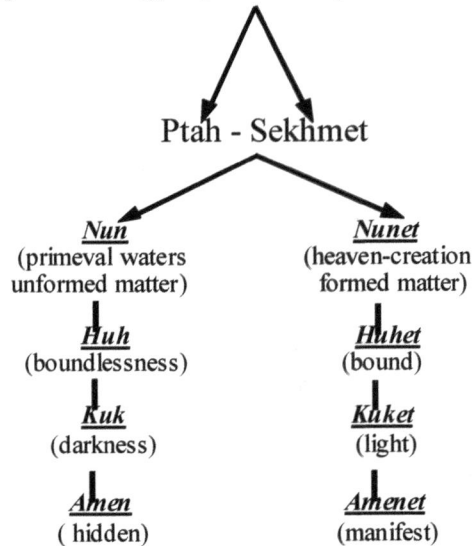

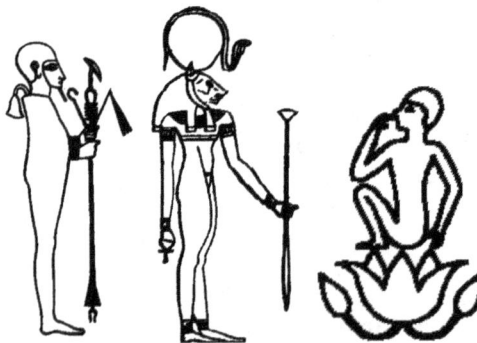

Ptah - Sekhmet

Nun (primeval waters unformed matter)	*Nunet* (heaven-creation formed matter)
Huh (boundlessness)	*Huhet* (bound)
Kuk (darkness)	*Kuket* (light)
Amen (hidden)	*Amenet* (manifest)

Ptah, Sekhmit and Nefertem

---

[13] See the Book Memphite Theology by Muata Ashby

The Theban Tradition

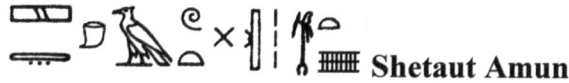

Shetaut Amun

The Mystery Teachings of the Wasetian Tradition are related to the Neterus known as Amun, Mut Khonsu. This temple and its related temples espoused the teachings of Creation, human origins and the path to spiritual enlightenment by means of the Supreme Being in the form of the god Amun or Amun-Ra. It tells of how Amun and his family, the Trinity of Amun, Mut and Khonsu, manage the Universe along with his Company of Gods and Goddesses. This Temple became very important in the early part of the New Kingdom Era.

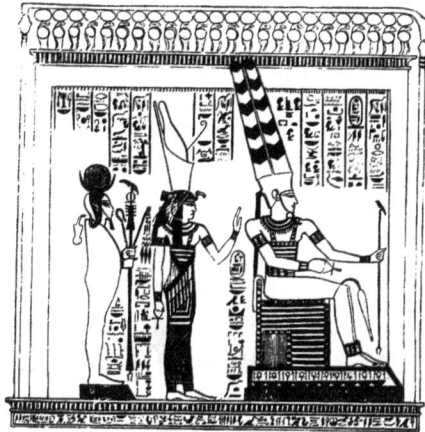

Below: The Trinity of Amun and the Company of Gods and Goddesses of Amun

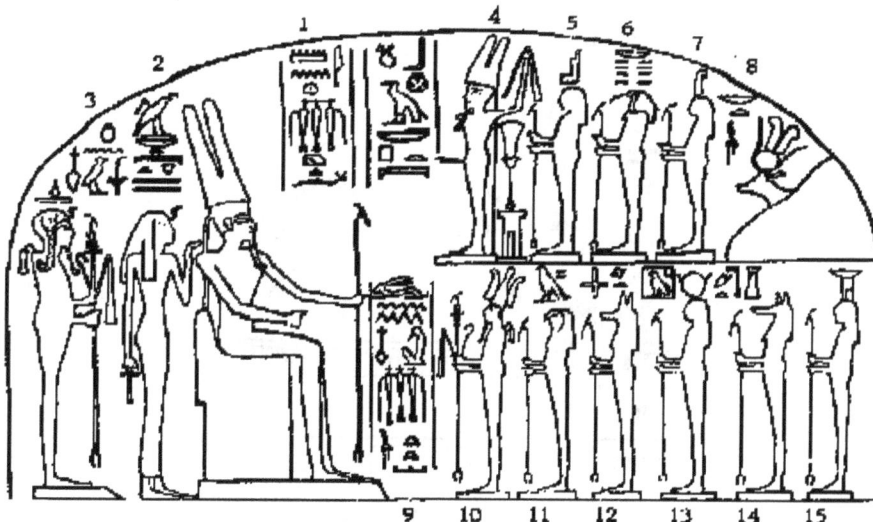

See the Book *Egyptian Yoga Vol. 2* for more on Amun, Mut and Khonsu by Muata Ashby

The Goddess Tradition

Shetaut Netrit

"Arat"

The hieroglyphic sign Arat means "Goddess." General, throughout ancient Kamit, the Mystery Teachings of the Goddess Tradition are related to the Divinity in the form of the Goddess. The Goddess was an integral part of all the Neterian traditions but special temples also developed around the worship of certain particular Goddesses who were also regarded as Supreme Beings in their own right. Thus as in other African religions, the goddess as well as the female gender were respected and elevated as the male divinities. The Goddess was also the author of Creation, giving birth to it as a great Cow. The following are the most important forms of the goddess.[14]

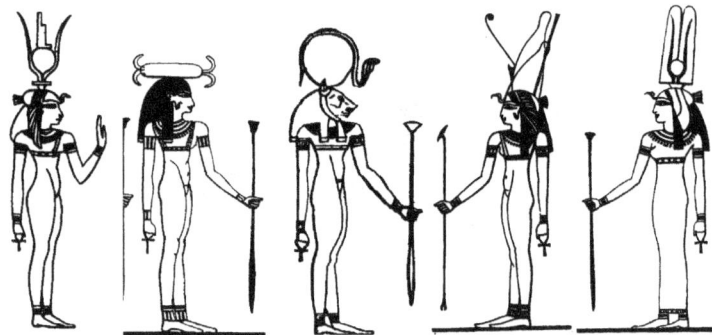

Aset, Net, Sekhmit, Mut, Hetheru

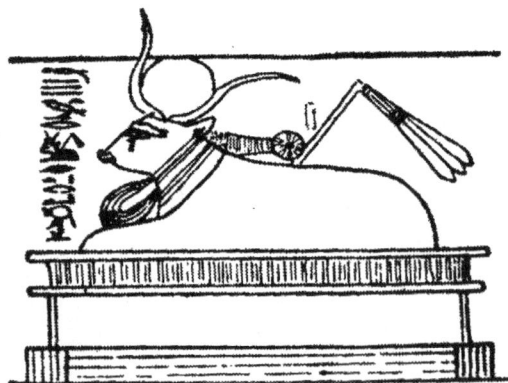

Mehurt ("The Mighty Full One")

---

[14] See the Books, *The Goddess Path, Mysteries of Isis, Glorious Light Meditation, Memphite Theology* and *Resurrecting Osiris* by Muata Ashby

The Asarian Tradition

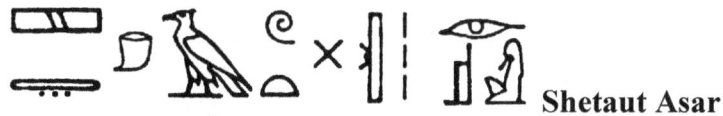 **Shetaut Asar**

This temple and its related temples espoused the teachings of Creation, human origins and the path to spiritual enlightenment by means of the Supreme Being in the form of the god Asar. It tells of how Asar and his family, the Trinity of Asar, Aset and Heru, manage the Universe and lead human beings to spiritual enlightenment and the resurrection of the soul. This Temple and its teaching were very important from the Pre-Dynastic era down to the Christian period. The Mystery Teachings of the Asarian Tradition are related to the Neterus known as: Asar, Aset, Heru (Osiris, Isis and Horus)

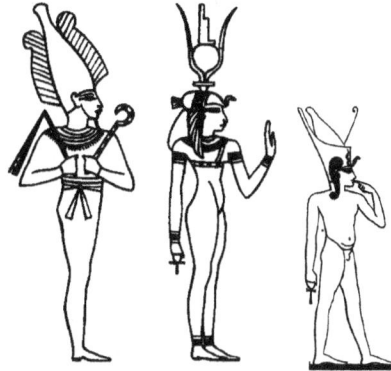

The tradition of Asar, Aset and Heru was practiced generally throughout the land of ancient Kamit. The centers of this tradition were the city of Abdu containing the Great Temple of Asar, the city of Pilak containing the Great Temple of Aset[15] and Edfu containing the Ggreat Temple of Heru.

---

[15] See the Book Resurrecting Osiris by Muata Ashby

The Aton Tradition

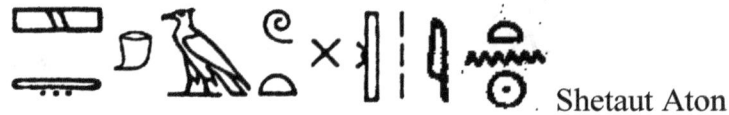 Shetaut Aton

This temple and its related temples espoused the teachings of Creation, human origins and the path to spiritual enlightenment by means of the Supreme Being in the form of the god Aton. It tells of how Aton with its dynamic life force created and sustains Creation. By recognizing Aton as the very substratum of all existence, human beings engage in devotional exercises and rituals and the study of the Hymns containing the wisdom teachings of Aton explaining that Aton manages the Universe and leads human beings to spiritual enlightenment and eternal life for the soul. This Temple and its teaching were very important in the middle New Kingdom Period. The Mystery Teachings of the Aton Tradition are related to the Neter Aton and its main exponent was the Sage King Akhnaton, who is depicted below with his family adoring the sundisk, symbol of the Aton.

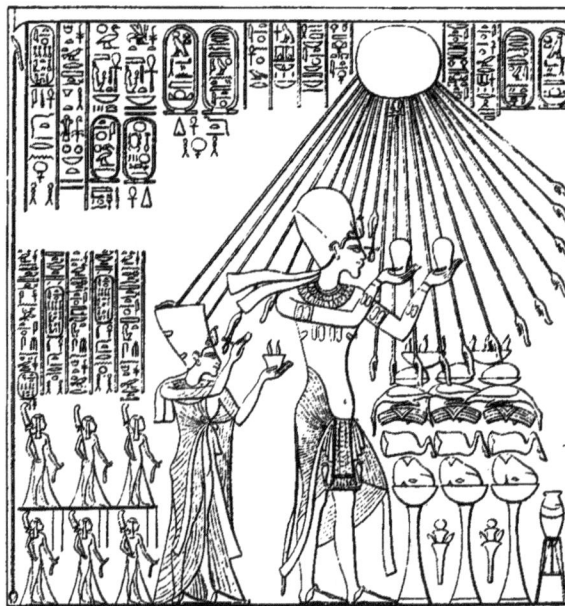

Akhnaton, Nefertiti and Daughters

For more on Atonism and the Aton Theology see the Essence of Atonism Lecture Series by Sebai Muata Ashby ©2001

The General Principles of Shetaut Neter
(Teachings Presented in the Kamitan scriptures)

1. The Purpose of Life is to Attain the Great Awakening-Enlightenment-Know thyself.

2. SHETAUT NETER enjoins the Shedy (spiritual investigation) as the highest endeavor of life.

3. SHETAUT NETER enjoins that it is the responsibility of every human being to promote order and truth.

4. SHETAUT NETER enjoins the performance of Selfless Service to family, community and humanity.

5. SHETAUT NETER enjoins the Protection of nature.

6. SHETAUT NETER enjoins the Protection of the weak and oppressed.

7. SHETAUT NETER enjoins the Caring for hungry.

8. SHETAUT NETER enjoins the Caring for homeless.

9. SHETAUT NETER enjoins the equality for all people.

10. SHETAUT NETER enjoins the equality between men and women.

11. SHETAUT NETER enjoins the justice for all.

12. SHETAUT NETER enjoins the sharing of resources.

13. SHETAUT NETER enjoins the protection and proper raising of children.

14. SHETAUT NETER enjoins the movement towards balance and peace.

The Forces of Entropy

In Neterian religion, there is no concept of "evil" as is conceptualized in Western Culture. Rather, it is understood that the forces of entropy are constantly working in nature to bring that which has been constructed by human hands to their original natural state. The serpent Apep (Apophis), who daily tries to stop Ra's boat of creation, is the symbol of entropy. This concept of entropy has been referred to as "chaos" by Western Egyptologists.

Apep

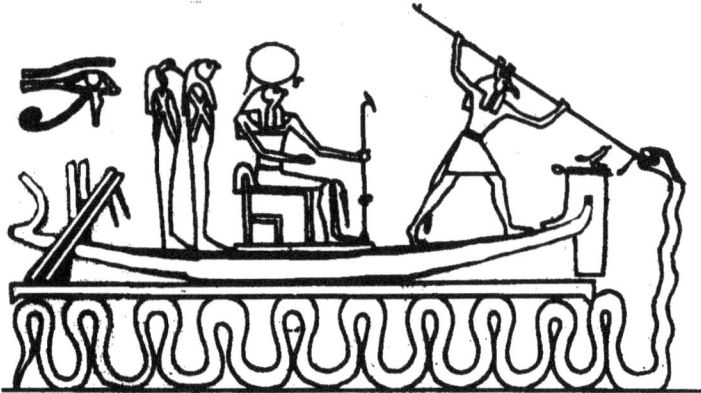

Above: Set protecting the boat of Ra from the forces of entropy (symbolized by the serpent Apep).

As expressed previously, in Neterian religion there is also no concept of a "devil" or "demon" as is conceived in the Judeo-Christian or Islamic traditions. Rather, it is understood that manifestations of detrimental situations and adversities arise as a result of unrighteous actions. These unrighteous actions are due to the "Setian" qualities in a human being. Set is the Neteru of egoism and the negative qualities which arise from egoism. Egoism is the idea of individuality based on identification with the body and mind only as being who one is. One has no deeper awareness of their deeper spiritual essence, and thus no understanding of their connectedness to all other objects (includes persons) in creation and the Divine Self. When the ego is under the control of the higher nature, it fights the forces of entropy (as above). However, when beset with ignorance, it leads to the degraded states of human existence. The vices (egoism, selfishness, extraverted ness, wonton sexuality (lust), jealousy, envy, greed, gluttony) are a result.

Set

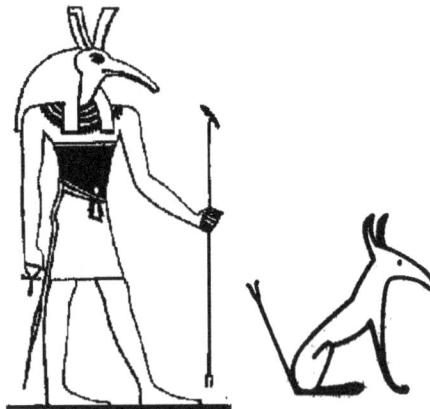

Set and the Set animal

The Great Awakening of Neterian Religion

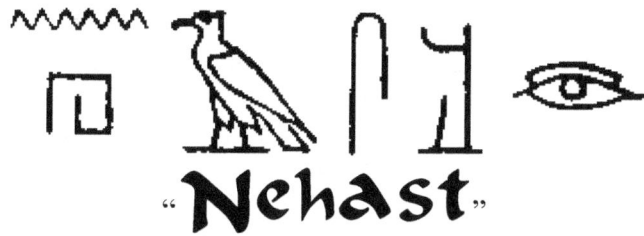

"Nehast"

Nehast means to "wake up," to Awaken to the higher existence. In the Prt m Hru Text it is said:

Nuk pa Neter aah Neter Ujah asha ren[16]

"I am that same God, the Supreme One, who has myriad of mysterious names."

The goal of all the Neterian disciplines is to discover the meaning of "Who am I?," to unravel the mysteries of life and to fathom the depths of eternity and infinity. This is the task of all human beings and it is to be accomplished in this very lifetime.

This can be done by learning the ways of the Neteru, emulating them and finally becoming like them, Akhus, (enlightened beings), walking the earth as giants and accomplishing great deeds such as the creation of the universe!

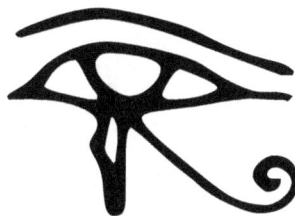

Udjat

The Eye of Heru is a quintessential symbol of awakening to Divine Consciousness, representing the concept of Nehast.

---

[16] (Prt M Hru 9:4)

The Cities in Ancient Egypt Where the Greek Philosophers Studied

The land of Ancient Egypt

Solon, Thales, Plato, Eudoxus and Pythagoras went to Egypt and consorted with the priests. Eudoxus they say, received instruction from Chonuphis of Memphis,* Solon from Sonchis of Sais,* and Pythagoras from Oeniphis of Heliopolis.*

–Plutarch (Greek historian c. 46-120 A.C.E.)

*(cities in Ancient Egypt-see below)

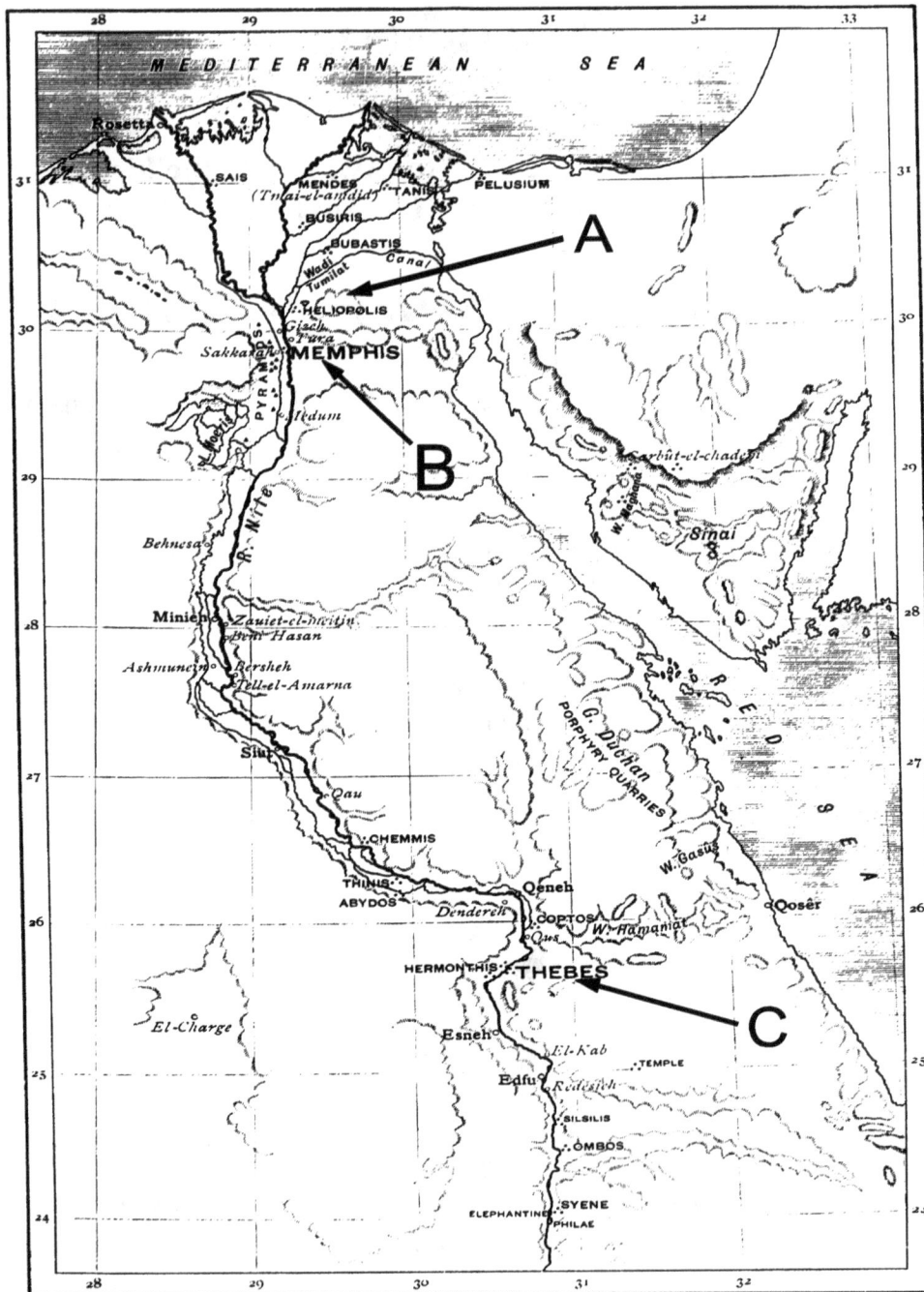

Key to the Map above: Egypt is located in the north-eastern corner of the African Continent. The cities wherein the theology of the Trinity of Amun-Ra-Ptah was developed were: A- Anu (Heliopolis), B-Hetkaptah (Memphis), and C-Waset (Thebes).

Sacred Scriptures of Shetaut Neter

The following scriptures represent the foundational scriptures of Kamitan culture. They may be divided into three categories: *Mythic Scriptures*, *Mystical Philosophy* and *Ritual Scriptures*, and *Wisdom Scriptures* (Didactic Literature).

MYTHIC SCRIPTURES Literature	Mystical (Ritual) Philosophy Literature	Wisdom Texts Literature
Shetaut Asar-Aset-Heru The Myth of Asar, Aset and Heru (Asarian Resurrection Theology) - Predynastic **Shetaut Atum-Ra** Anunian Theology Predynastic **Shetaut Net/Aset/Hetheru** Saitian Theology – Goddess Spirituality Predynastic **Shetaut Ptah** Memphite Theology Predynastic **Shetaut Amun** Theban Theology Predynastic	**Pyramid Texts** (c. 5500 B.C.E.-3800 B.C.E.) **Coffin Texts** (c. 2040 B.C.E.-1786 B.C.E.) **Papyrus Texts** (c. 1580 B.C.E.-Roman Period)[17] Books of Coming Forth By Day Example of famous papyri: Papyrus of Any Papyrus of Hunefer Papyrus of Kenna Greenfield Papyrus, Etc.	**Wisdom Texts** (c. 3,000 B.C.E. – Ptolemaic Period) Precepts of Ptahotep Instructions of Any Instructions of Amenemope Etc. Maat Declarations Literature (All Periods) Songs of the Blind Harper

---

[17] After 1570 B.C.E they would evolve into a more unified text, the Egyptian Book of the Dead.

Medu Neter

"Medu Neter"

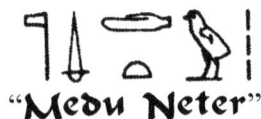

The teachings of the Neterian Traditions are conveyed in the scriptures of the Neterian Traditions. These are recorded in the Medu Neter script.

Old Period Hieroglyphic Script

Above: A section from the pyramid of Teti in Sakkara Egypt, known as the "Pyramid Texts" (Early Dynastic Period) showing the cross

The Medu Neter was used through all periods by Priests and priestesses – mostly used in monumental inscriptions such as the Pyramid texts, Obelisks, temple inscriptions, etc. – since Pre-Dynastic times. It is the earliest form of writing in known history.

Hekau, Medu Neter and Shetitu

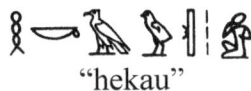

"hekau"

The concept of the divine word or *Hekau,* is an extremely important part of Ancient Egyptian religion and is instructive in the study of all African religion. The only difference between Ancient Egyptian religion and other African religions in this area was the extensive development of the "written word." As explained earlier, the word religion is translated as Shetaut Neter in the Ancient African language of Kamit.

Shetitu

This Shetaut (mysteries- rituals, wisdom, philosophy) about the Neter (Supreme Being) are related in the *Shetitu* or writings related to the hidden teaching. And those writings are referred to as *Medu Neter* or "Divine Speech," the writings of the god Djehuti (Ancient Egyptian god of the divine word) – also refers to any hieroglyphic texts or inscriptions generally. The term Medu Neter makes use of a special hieroglyph, , which means "*medu*" or "staff - walking stick-speech." This means that speech is the support for the Divine, . Thus, just as the staff supports an elderly person, the hieroglyphic writing (the word) is a prop (staff) which sustains the Divine in the realm of time and space. That is, the Divine writings contain the wisdom which enlightens us about to the Divine, *Shetaut Neter.*

If Medu Neter is mastered then the spiritual aspirant becomes Maakheru or true of thought, word and deed, that is, purified in body, mind and soul. The symbol medu is static while the symbol of Kheru is dynamic.

This term (Maakheru) uses the glyph kheru is a rudder – oar (rowing), symbol of voice, meaning that purification occurs when the righteous movement of the word, when it is used (rowing-movement) to promote virtue, order, peace, harmony and truth. So Medu Neter is the potential word and Maa kheru is the perfected word.

The hieroglyphic texts (Medu Neter) become (Maakheru) useful in the process of religion when they are used as hekau - the Ancient Egyptian "Words of Power" when the word is Hesi, chanted and Shmai- sung and thereby one performs **or** Dua or worship of the Divine. The divine word allows the speaker to control the gods and goddesses, i.e. the cosmic forces. This concept is really based on the idea that human beings are higher order beings if they learn about the nature of the universe and elevate themselves through virtue and wisdom.

The General Principles of Shetaut Neter

15. The Purpose of Life is to Attain the Great Awakening-Enlightenment-Know thyself.
16. SHETAUT NETER enjoins the Shedy (spiritual investigation) as the highest endeavor of life.
17. SHETAUT NETER enjoins the responsibility of every human being is to promote order and truth.
18. SHETAUT NETER enjoins the performance of Selfless Service to family, community and humanity.
19. SHETAUT NETER enjoins the Protection of nature.
20. SHETAUT NETER enjoins the Protection of the weak and oppressed.
21. SHETAUT NETER enjoins the Caring for hungry.
22. SHETAUT NETER enjoins the Caring for homeless.
23. SHETAUT NETER enjoins the equality for all people.
24. SHETAUT NETER enjoins the equality between men and women.
25. SHETAUT NETER enjoins the justice for all.
26. SHETAUT NETER enjoins the sharing of resources.
27. SHETAUT NETER enjoins the protection and proper raising of children.
28. SHETAUT NETER enjoins the movement towards balance and peace.

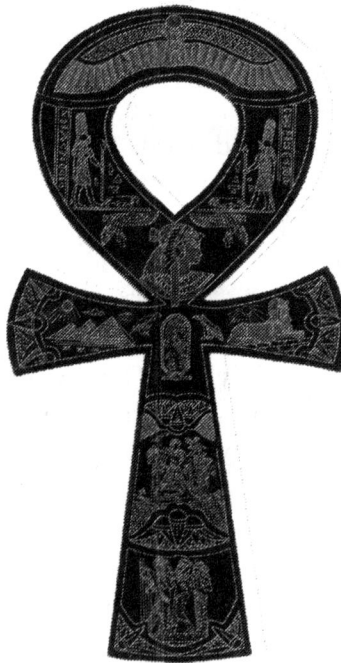

THE PURPOSE AND GOAL OF NETERIAN THEATER

IN present day western theater the purpose is often to provide entertainment for an audience and to provide the unique form of pleasure that can be experienced by an actor when he or she performs. For some people the act of acting is a form of art wherein they express a sentiment or an idea through the performance of a play. For others it is an opportunity to gratify their egoistic desire to be lauded over, praised and looked up to.

In Neterian Theater the objective is not just to entertain or provide an opportunity for personal aggrandizement. In Neterian Theater the purpose is to provide a venue for the expert and profuse practice of a religious ritual. The ritual is the performance of a myth and the myth is the special language of a spiritual teaching through which the feeling and experience of the Neterian gods and goddesses can be communed with. If such a communion were to occur it would be possible to not only act out parts, taking on the costumes and names of characters in the divine plays but also it would be possible to become one with those characters, the gods and goddesses. Then, knowing and experiencing as they do, the Neterian actors also become one with the source of their knowing and experiencing which is the Supreme and all-encompassing being.

So the ultimate goal in Neterian Theater is to make the Neterian Myth effective, that is, a reality in the mind and heart of the actor. So the Neterian ritual, for instance, of the Pert m Hru or "Book of the Dead" is to make the myth of Asar, Aset and Heru come alive, therefore, becoming one with them. Each Neterian Tradition has special myth which tell the story of the origins of Creation and the means to discover the ultimate mysteries of life. The practice of ritual is a theatrical performance of the myth that allows the participants to live the myth. So the myth is not an occurrence of the past, for people of the past alone. It is a reenactment of transcendental truths that are true in the past, present and future.

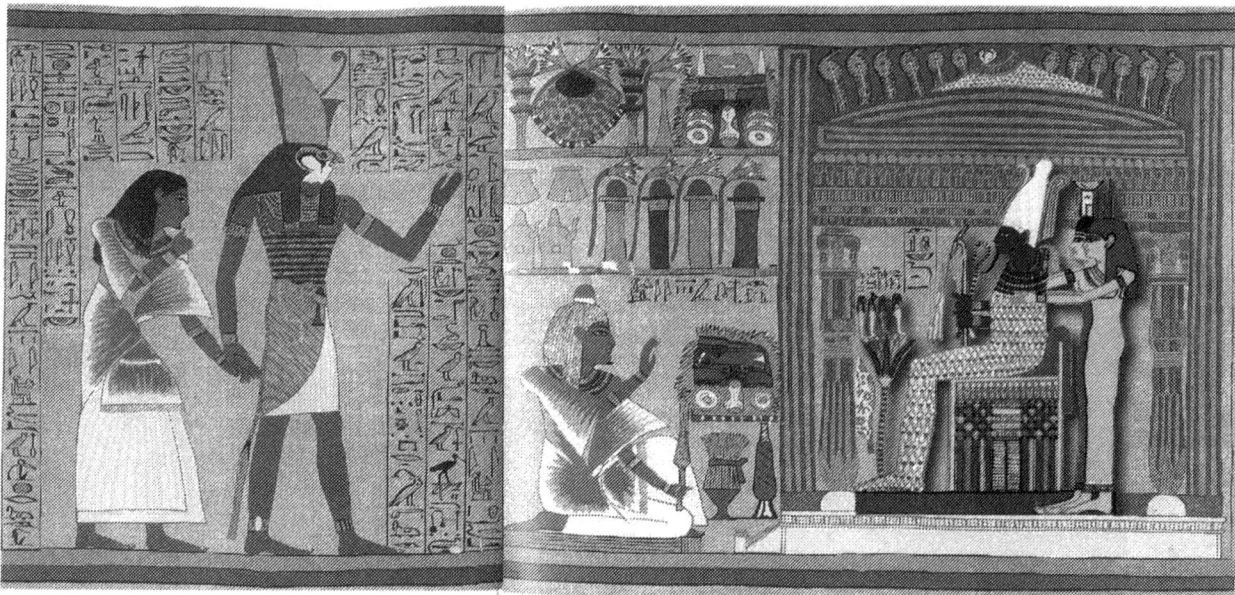

Above: Scene from the ritual play of the Per m Hru of Ani. Ani enacts the ideal of being pure and being led by Heru to the inner shrine wherein he meets Asar.

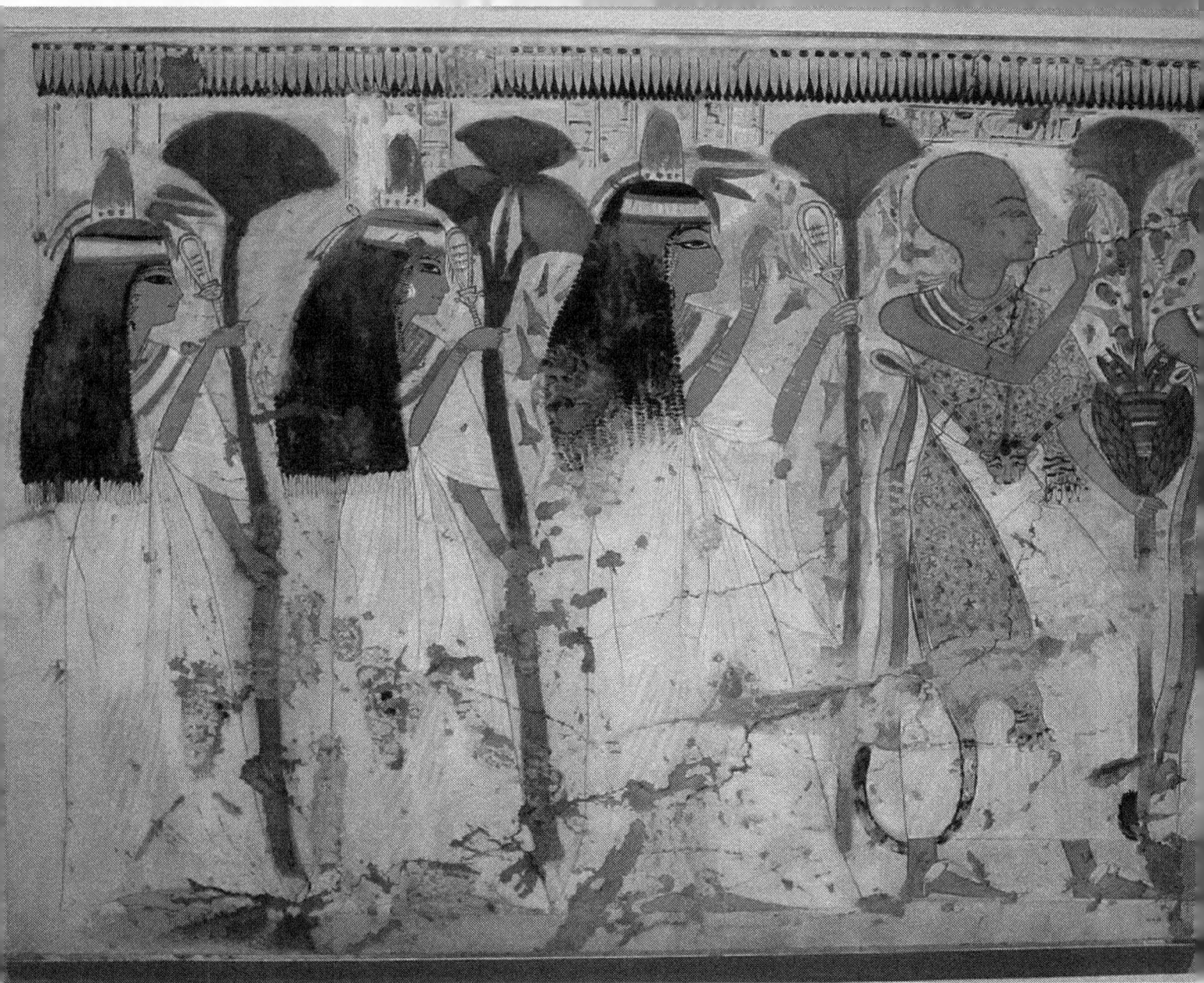

Above: the priests and priestesses make offerings to the Divine.

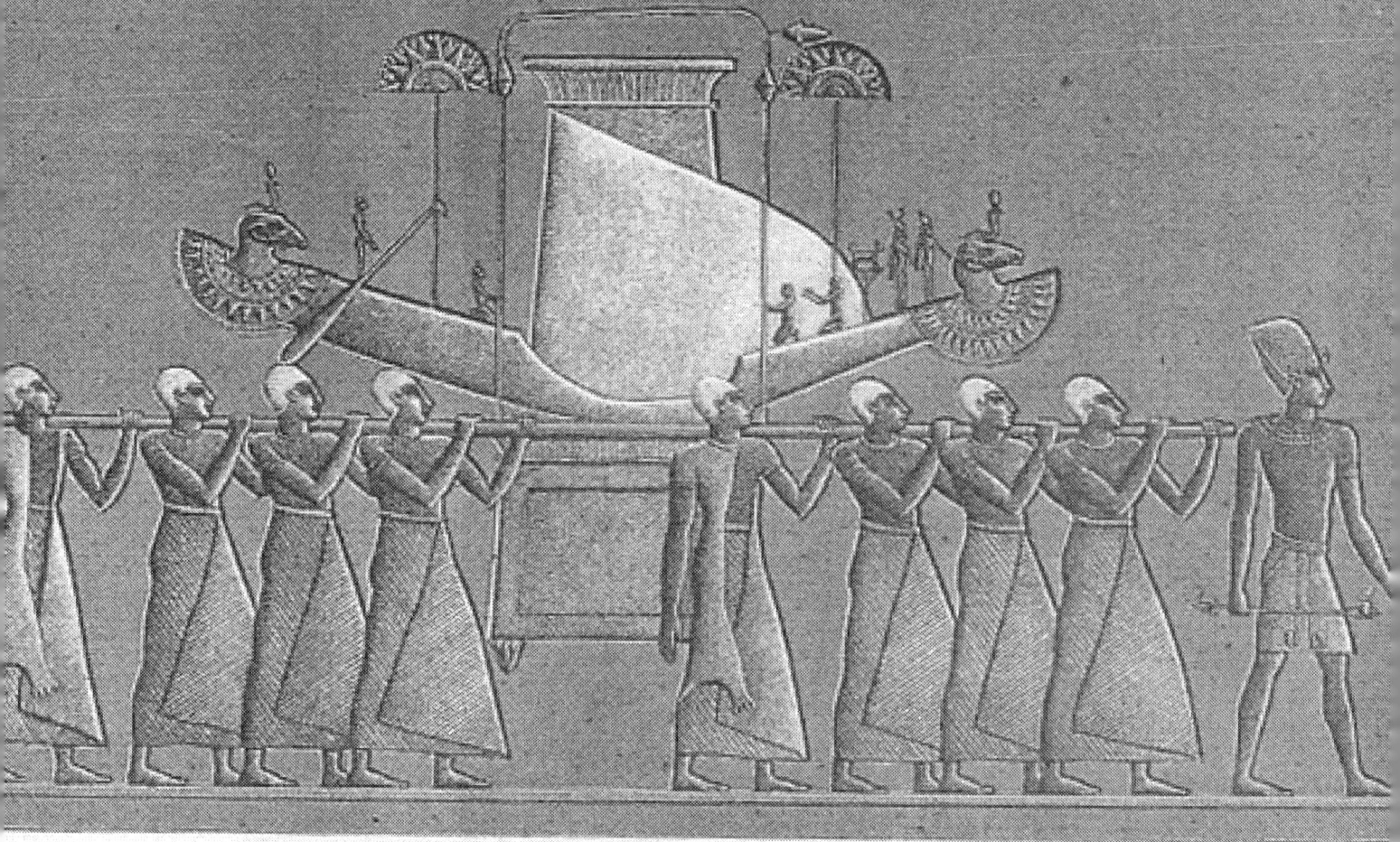

Above: the priests carry out the ritual of carrying the divine boat of Amun.

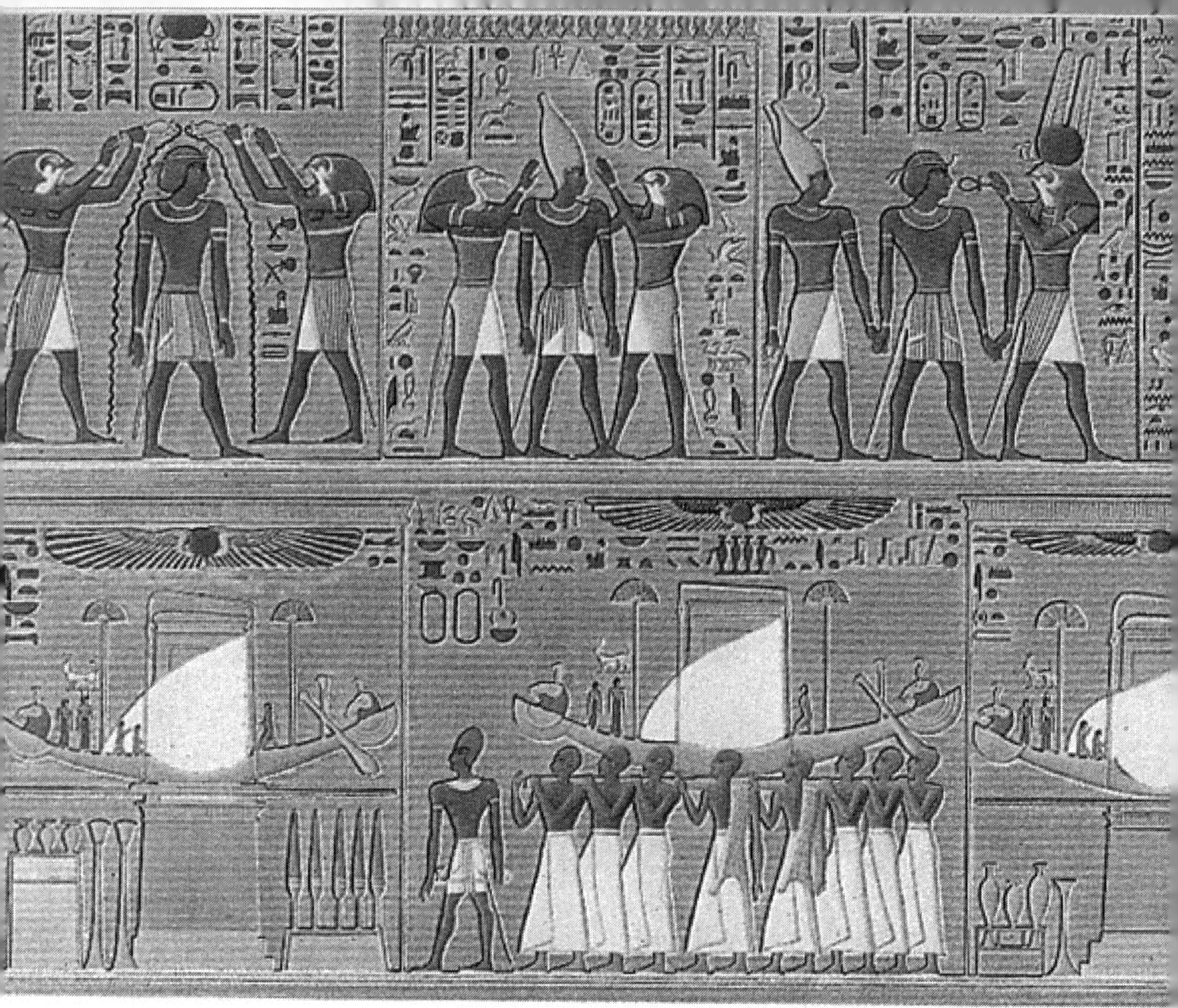

Philip Arrhidaeus, successor of Alexander, a Greek, in depicted in Red (From the Napoleonic Expedition)

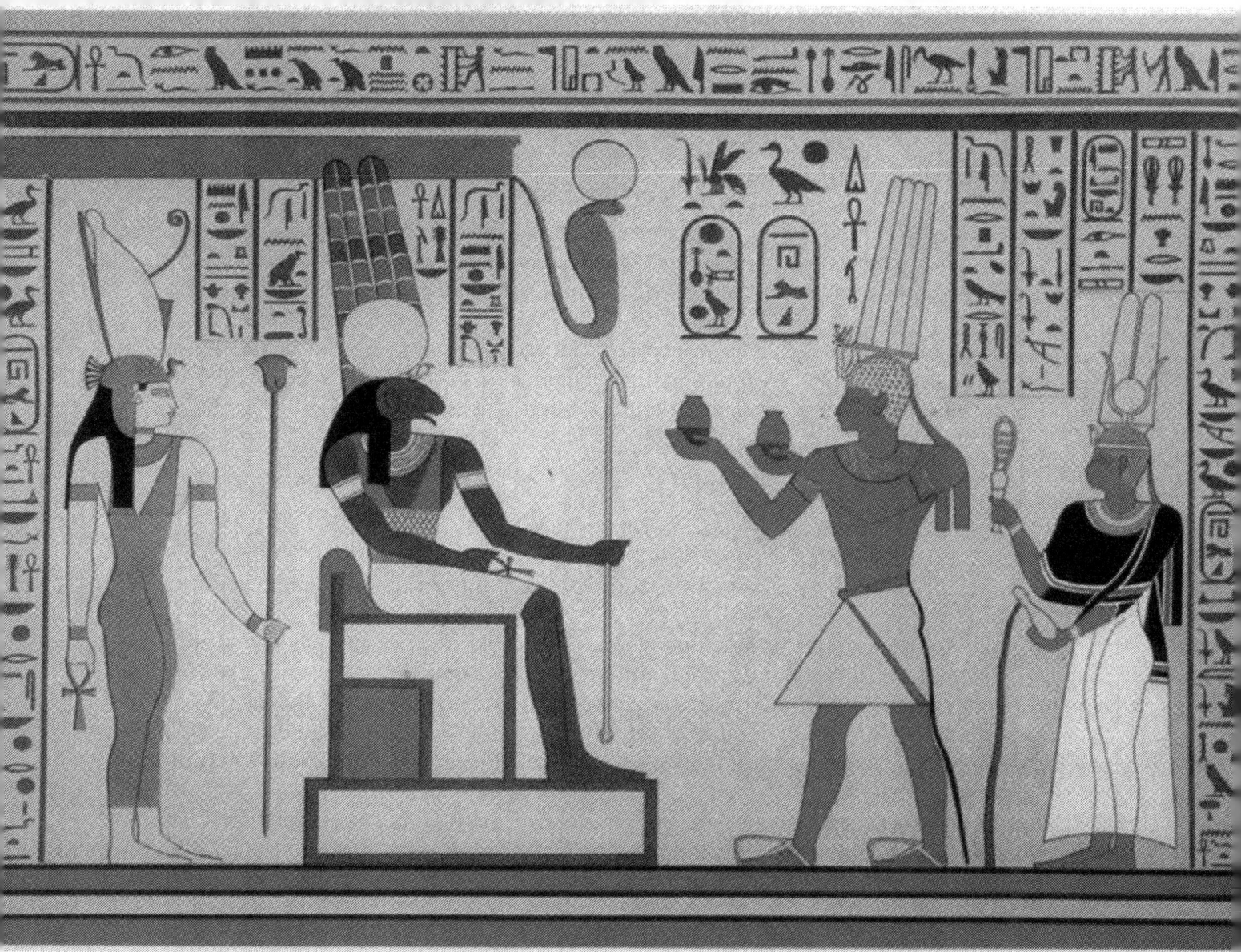

Nubian King Taharka and the Queen offering to Amun (blue) and Mut (colored in yellow) depicted as a red Egyptians. 7th cent BCE

PLAY STRUCTURE AND GRAMMAR

The play has been configured for the proscenium stage which is still the most common form of theater. It requires four main cast members. The play is approximately 45-60 minutes in length and it is designed for community groups as well as professional theater productions.

Many important elements have been incorporated into the grammatical structure of the play. The tone and meter of Ancient Egyptian writing is unique in and of itself. In contrast to Western grammar, the basic structure of Ancient Egyptian writing is as follows:

1- particle
    2- the verb
        3- the subject
            4- the direct object
                5- adverbial modifiers (prepositional phrases, indirect object, etc.)

I have tried to incorporate this structure wherever possible so as to give the play a closer feel to the original text. Also, Ancient Egyptian writing often had a poetic quality and very often used punning. Punning, or a play on words, sometimes on different senses of the same word and sometimes on the similar sense or sound of different words, was used to indicate deeper, more subtle meanings to the writing, like a hidden teaching underneath the surface story or word.

Thus I have incorporated rhyme into the structure of the play but only for those characters who are evolved or who experience an elevated state of consciousness. Thus, Hetheru does not speak poetically when she is under the delusion, but does so when she becomes enlightened as to her true nature.

Other elements included in this play include Kamitan terms. These were known as Hekau or words of power. Words of power were and are used to promote and affirm a teaching, and the understanding of that teaching, as well as to engender positive vibrations in one's own mind as well as the environment. Thus, at the end of the play, there is a reenactment of the ancient ritual of Hetheru and many Hekau are used.

Another important element in the structure of the play is the relationship between Djehuti and Hetheru. This is known as the teacher-disciple relationship. From ancient times aspiring students of spiritual philosophy have sought out spiritual preceptors, Sebais, priests and priestesses, gurus, etc., to teach them the subtleties of mysticism. Thus, for the first time in history we have such a relationship being played out which is akin to the relationship between the characters of Krishna and Arjuna in India, or Jesus and John the Baptist in Christianity. This aspect of the story will be discussed in more detail in the Gloss at the end of this book. Ultimately, this is a story with perennial implications. It should be studied again and again and practiced in one's life. This is the deeper purpose of the play, to remind us of a higher truth, even though we are caught up in the illusions of life.

Perhaps the most important element I have tried to incorporate into the structure of the play is the glimpse into Ancient Egyptian mythology and its mystical as well as societal implications.

Maat philosophy is the unique gift from Africa to the world, and it has influenced other cultures, such as Greek culture and in turn, modern Western culture as well. But ultimately, The Enlightenment of Hetheru is the saga of self-discovery, the quest which every human being faces on an individual level. Thus, it has personal and universal applications, in all periods of history.

This story is also tied into a greater and more profound philosophy as well, is the philosophy of Yoga. Towards the end of the play, Djehuti leads Hetheru on a guided meditation as a means of awakening her deeper memories. The actual hieroglyphic text upon which this play is based prescribes that a meditation is to be performed following the performance of the ritual (play) and/or the reading of the text. Thus, the yogic mystical discipline of Yoga Meditation is an integral part of the original story, and is here reproduced and updated for our times. This text appears to be the first documented text describing a formal meditation discipline in human history.

WHAT IS YOGA PHILOSOPHY?

Since a complete treatise on the theory and practice of yoga would require several volumes, only a basic outline will be given here.

When we look out upon the world, we are often baffled by the multiplicity, which constitutes the human experience. What do we really know about this experience? Many scientific disciplines have developed over the last two hundred years for the purpose of discovering the mysteries of nature, but this search has only engendered new questions about the nature of existence. Yoga is a discipline or way of life designed to promote the physical, mental and spiritual development of the human being. It leads a person to discover the answers to the most important questions of life such as "Who am I?" "Why am I here?" and "Where am I going?"

The literal meaning of the word YOGA is to "YOKE" or to "LINK" back. The implication is: to link back to the original source, the original essence, that which transcends all mental and intellectual attempts at comprehension, but which is the essential nature of everything in CREATION. While in the strict or dogmatic sense, Yoga philosophy and practice is a separate discipline from religion, yoga and religion have been linked at many points throughout history. Religion has three aspects, myth, ritual and mysticism. Myth and ritual relate to the folk expression of religion, whereas mysticism relates to that movement of self-discovery that transcends all worldly concepts. The Ancient Egyptian theater belongs to the ritual level of religion because it affords its practitioners to transition from just hearing the myth to acting it out and thereby feeling or experiencing it and moving towards a mystical awakening. Mysticism allows any person in any religion to discover that the same Supreme Being is being worshipped by all under different names and forms, and by different means. In a manner of speaking, Yoga as a discipline may be seen as a non-sectarian transpersonal science or practice to promote spiritual development and harmony of mind and body thorough mental and physical disciplines including meditation, psycho-physical exercises, and performing action with the correct attitude.

The disciplines of Yoga fall under five major categories. These are Yoga of Wisdom, Yoga of Devotional Love, Yoga of Meditation, Tantric Yoga and Yoga of Selfless Action. Within these categories there are subsidiary forms which are part of the main disciplines. The important point to remember is that all aspects of yoga can and should be used in an integral fashion to effect an efficient and harmonized spiritual movement in the practitioner. Therefore, while there may be an area of special emphasis, other elements are bound to become part of the yoga program as needed. For example, while a yogin may place emphasis on the yoga of devotion, they will also be led to practice wisdom yoga, action yoga and meditation yoga along with the wisdom studies.

While it is true that yogic practices may be found in religion, strictly speaking, yoga is neither a religion nor a philosophy. It should be thought of more as a way of life or discipline for promoting greater fullness and experience of life. Those who wanted more out of life developed yoga at the dawn of history. These special men and women wanted to discover the true origins of creation and of themselves. Therefore, they set out to explore the vast reaches of consciousness within themselves. They are sometimes referred to as "Seers", "Sages", etc. Awareness or consciousness can only be increased when the mind is in a state of peace and harmony. Thus, the disciplines of meditation (which are part of Yoga), and wisdom (the philosophical teachings for understanding reality as it is) are the primary means to controlling the mind and allowing the individual to mature psychologically and spiritually.

The teachings, which were practiced in the Ancient Egyptian temples, were the same ones later intellectually defined into a literary form by the Indian Sages of Vedanta and Yoga. This was discussed in my book *Egyptian Yoga: The Philosophy of Enlightenment* and is further elaborated in the book *African Origins of Civilization, Religion and Yoga Spirituality*. The Indian Mysteries of Yoga and Vedanta represent an unfolding and intellectual exposition of the Egyptian Mysteries. Also, Gnostic Christianity or Christianity before Roman Catholicism originated in Ancient Egypt, and was also based on the Ancient Egyptian Mysteries. (See the book *Mystical Journey from Jesus to Christ* by Muata Ashby)

The question is how to accomplish these seemingly impossible tasks? How to transform yourself and realize the deepest mysteries of existence? How to discover "Who am I?" This is the mission of Yoga Philosophy and the purpose of yogic practices. Yoga does not seek to convert or impose religious beliefs on any one. Ancient Egypt was the source of civilization and the source of religion and Yoga. Therefore, all systems of religion (practiced in its complete form) and mystical spirituality can coexist harmoniously within these teachings when they are correctly understood.

The goal of yoga is to promote integration of the mind-body-spirit complex, in order to produce optimal health of the human being. This is accomplished through mental and physical exercises, which promote the free flow of spiritual energy by reducing mental complexes caused by ignorance. There are two roads which human beings can follow, the path of wisdom and the other of ignorance. The path of the masses is generally the path of ignorance, which leads them into negative situations, thoughts and deeds. These in turn lead to ill health and sorrow in life. The other road is based on wisdom and it leads to health, true happiness and enlightenment.

Therefore, the work of Ancient Egyptian theater had two purposes, to entertain and to enlighten the soul. Thus, we owe a debt of gratitude to the Sages who composed these myths and the philosophy behind them. They were not created just for our entertainment, but for conveying to us various teachings which are best expressed in a dramatic form, teachings related to our spiritual journey of life. Thus, the original theater, which produced the mystery plays performed in the Ancient Egyptian temple more than five thousand years ago, had a spiritual and educational purpose, and this potential still exists, today, as it did in the past. It is a forgotten art that needs to be revived. Otherwise, theater was degraded to the status of an entertainment instrument, serving not the intellect and heart, but the ego of a human being.

Images From the Temples of Goddess Hetheru

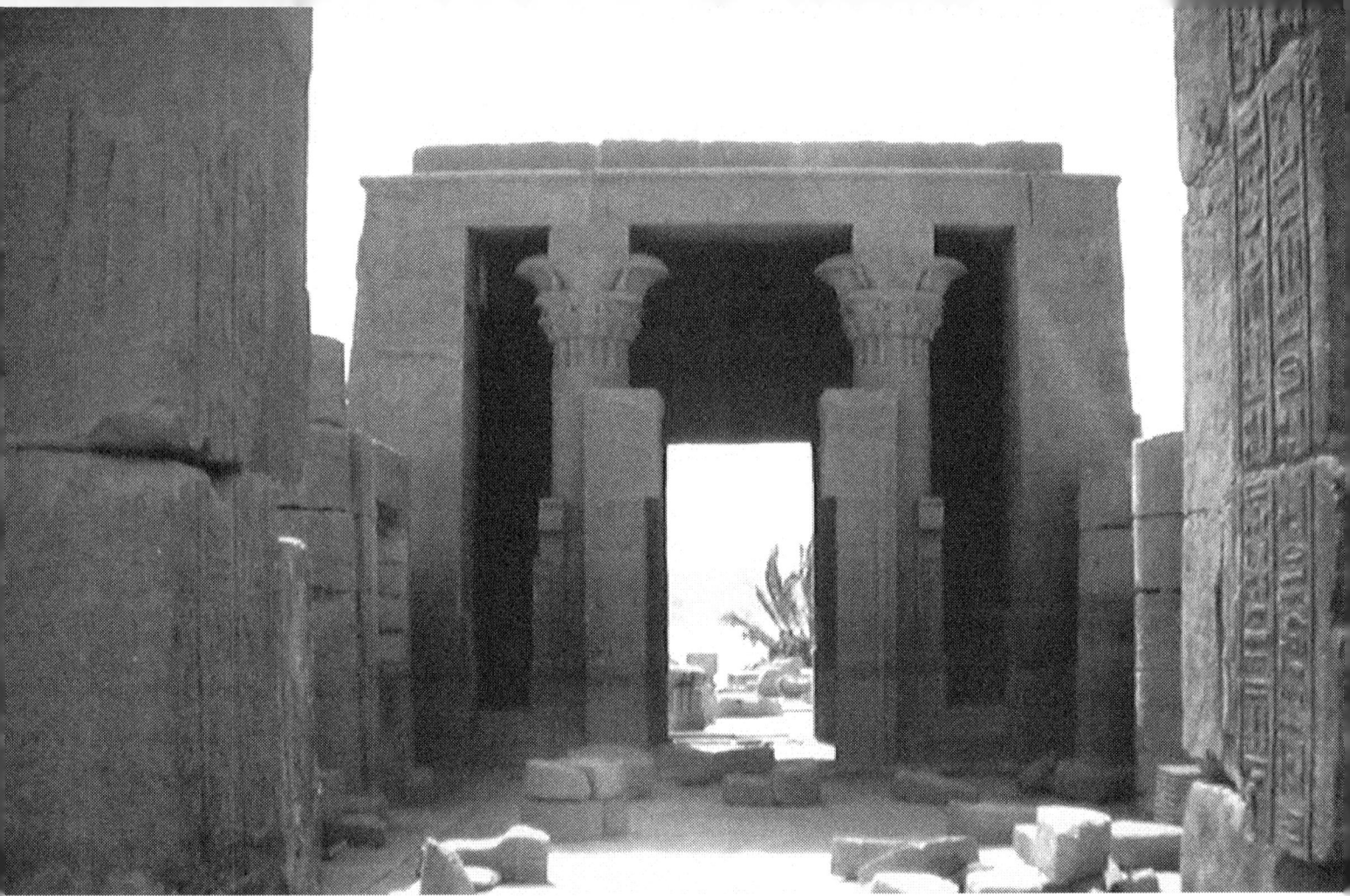

Above: Chapel of Hetheru at the Aset Temple complex in south Egypt (Aswan)

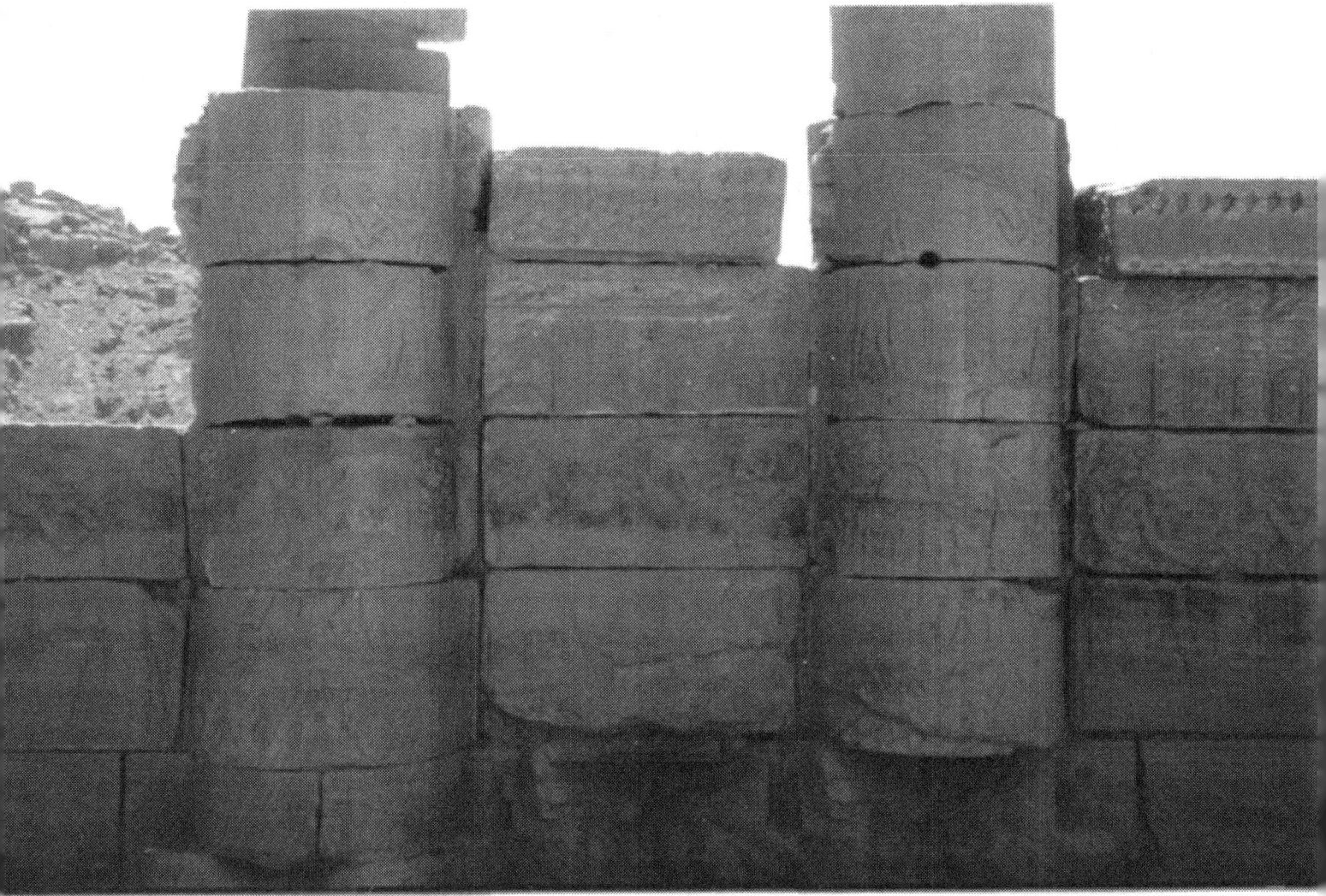

Above: Wall section of the Chapel of Hetheru (above) at the Aset Temple complex in south Egypt (Aswan) with a version of the story of the Enlightenment of Hetheru.

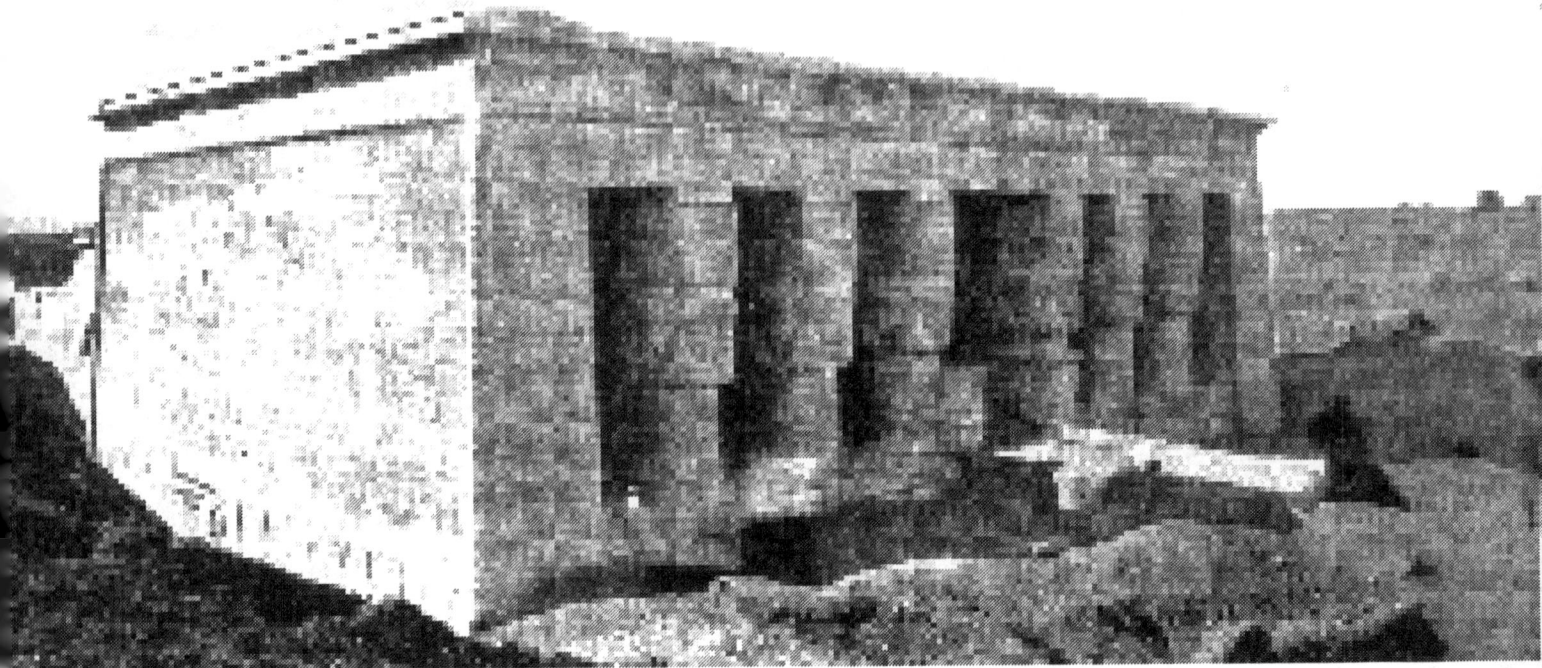

Right: Temple of Hetheru at Dendera, Kmt (Egypt)

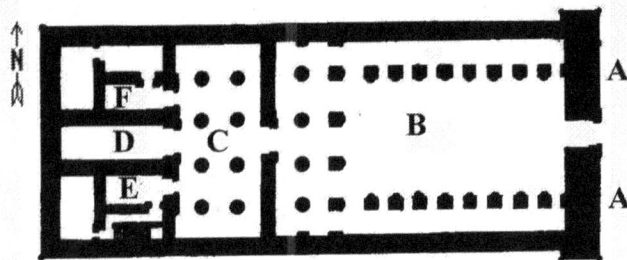

Above: A diagram of the Temple of Amun-Ra at Karnak, Egypt, showing (A) the open court and Pylons, (B) the Peristyle Hall (columns around the perimeter and open in center), (C) the Hypostyle Hall (covered area with many columns), (D) the Chapel of Amun (Holy of Holies), (E) the Chapel of Mut, (F) the Chapel of Khons.

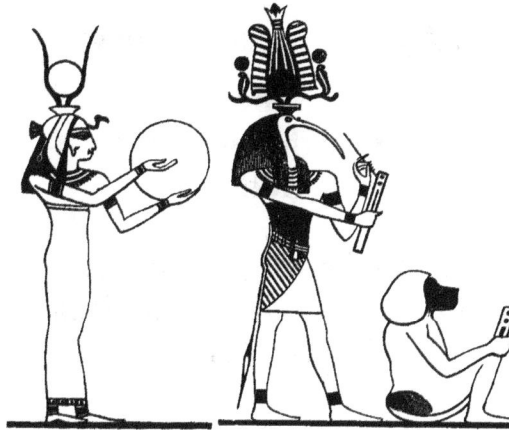

Left: The goddess Hetheru as a woman.

Right: Forms of the god Djehuti as an Ibis-headed man and as a Baboon.

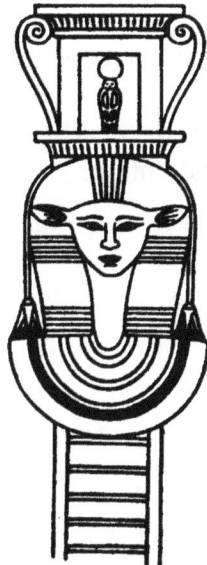

Above: A line art reproduction of a sistrum-column from the Temple of Hetheru in Egypt.

The Production
The
Enlightenment
Of Hetheru

An Ancient Egyptian Play
Adaptation of the original Kamitan texts by
Muata Ashby

Ancient Kamitan Terms and Ancient Greek Terms

In keeping with the spirit of the culture of Kamitan spirituality, in this volume we will use the Kamitan names for the divinities through which we will bring forth the Philosophy of the Kamitanism (Ancient Egyptian religion and myth). Therefore, the Greek name Osiris will be converted back to the Kamitan (Ancient Egyptian) Asar (Ausar), the Greek Isis to Aset (Auset), the Greek Nephthys to Nebthet, Anubis to Anpu or Apuat, Hathor to Hetheru, Thoth or Hermes to Djehuti, etc. (see the table below) Further, the term Ancient Egypt will be used interchangeably with "Kemit" ("Kamit"), or "Ta-Meri," as these were the terms used by the Ancient Egyptians to refer to their land and culture.

CHARACTER LIST IN ALPHABETICAL ORDER

1. CHOIR-CROWD- VICTIMS
2. DEMON #1
3. DEMON #2
4. DJEHUTI AS BABOON
5. DJEHUTI AS IBIS headed man
6. GEB
7. HETHERU
8. HETHERU AS LIONESS
9. HETHERU AS WOMAN
10. KAMITAN #1
11. KAMITAN #2
12. KAMITAN #3
13. KAMITAN #4
14. KAMITAN #5
15. KAMITAN #6
16. KAMITAN #7
17. KAMITAN #8
18. KAMITAN #9
19. KAMITANS
20. LIONESS
21. MAAT
22. NARRATOR
23. NUN
24. RA
25. SCRIBE

SCENE 1: RA AND THE PEOPLE

(LIGHTS COME UP ON THE PALACE OF RA IN THE CITY OF ANU. THE BACKGROUND
SHOULD SHOW A BUILDING AND IN THE DISTANCE THE SPHINX AND PYRAMIDS.)
(**RA** SITS ON A THRONE AND AT HIS SIDE IS HIS DAUGHTER MAAT- FACING THE
AUDIENCE a man with a writing pallet enters the stage and walks to the
front and begins to speak)

SCRIBE
I am a scribe of the venerable Lord Ra to do a noble task.
I learned and recorded this story in the tradition
of days past.

Many thousands of years ago the Lord of Lords and King of Kings, Ra
created the world and everything it.
He created everything in the universe but most beautiful of all things
is the beautiful land of Kamit.

As a righteous Monarch he watched over us as King. He commanded his
daughter Maat establish order and peace and justice in all the land,
to bring harmony to all things.

RA
Dearest daughter of mine, I charge you with the duty of establisher
and sustainer of the laws of righteousness in the world.
You will be the example for all who want to live by justice and truth
and allow goodness to unfurl.

If anyone disobeys your teachings, then they will experience pain and
suffering, for no one who goes against the laws of nature will find
peace or happiness by wrongdoing.

MAAT
Dearest Father mine, I accept your commission and from this day forth,
I will establish myself on the path of good thought.
Everyone who follows me will surely discover,
that righteous actions do bring order all over.

All who will follow my teachings will find the bright light of hetep -
peace- the coveted inner peace of the Divine.

(**RA** AND MAAT EXIT - MAAT AND HETHOR CAN
BE PLAYED BY THE SAME)

NARRATOR
For many thousands of years the law of the land was righteousness and
all people observed its principles.
There was joy, peace and happiness for everyone and a paradise indeed
on earth it was for everyone who followed its fundamentals.

(Two Egyptians walk in from opposite
sides of the stage. One is talking to
him/herself and the other one over
hears and interrupts.)

KAMITAN #8
(distressed-shaking head)

I do not know what to do! I really do not know what to do!

KAMITAN #9
(concerned)

Pardon me, I heard you say something just now. Is there some problem? You seem very distressed.

KAMITAN #8
(Worried and agitated)
This year my crops have not done well. I fear that my family will go hungry and that I will lose my home.

KAMITAN #9
(With a reassuring smile)

Please do not fear such calamities, for Ra takes care of those who follow Maat.

KAMITAN #8
What do you mean? I acted righteously and performed my duty but even so, misfortune has fallen upon me.
Anyway, why should you care about my misfortune. You are not even from our province?

KAMITAN #9
How can it be possible for Ra to leave us in our time of need? Does the sun ever cease to shine?
Does the air ever cease to bring the breath of life?
Fear not, I tell you because I too have seen misfortune and as surely as I stand here, I tell you that Ra takes care of all who follow Maat!

KAMITAN #8
Dear sir, your words are high minded and inspiring but I need help right now!

KAMITAN #9
(continuing)
Indeed. Help you shall have. I count myself as a fortunate follower of Maat and I am duty bound to help you in your time of need. I will share with you what I have and neither you nor your family will go hungry or lose your home.

KAMITAN #8
(Joyfully)
Truly is this an example of Maat! For one human being so caring for another is a sight to behold. I am lifted and heartened by your words of truth speaking, and my faith is reaffirmed in the glory of the Divine!

(EGYPTIANS #8-9 LEAVE STAGE AS NARRATOR
SPEAKS. EGYPTIANS #1-2 ENTER AND ACT AS
IF THEY ARE TALKING TO EACH OTHER.)

SCRIBE (O.S.)

Ra is the Creator of the universe.
He is the very source of all that exists.

Ra was the King of Kamit in the most ancient of times.
He ruled for thousands of years and the people loved and respected him as one Divine.

In time however, people became arrogant and prideful.
They forgot who had created and sustains the world, making all life possible.
What happened next is the story of Hetheru and Djehuti.
This story is a story of tragedy and pain and suffering but also one of victory and ultimate glory.

So listen carefully and you will learn,
the lessons of life and of how not to let the soul burn!

(WHEN THE NARRATOR FINISHES EGYPTIANS
1-2 BEGIN TO SPEAK OUT LOUD.)

KAMITAN #1
(egoistically)

I was there my dear. I went to the party of nobles and it was divine. I never enjoyed my self so much before.

KAMITAN #2

You are right! Those silly priests and priestesses are always telling us that we must pay homage to the gods and goddesses and practice Maat in order to be happy.

KAMITAN #1

(chuckling)
I pay homage to the host of the party!

KAMITAN #2

I agree! What do we need gods and goddesses for anyway? We waste our time going to the temples, and for what?

KAMITAN #1

Indeed! Not only time wasted but offerings as well.
Last week I gave a whole loaf of bread to the temple. I don't see the point.

KAMITAN #2

Yes. Last week I gave the temple a quarter of the
crops that I brought to the market. Why should that be?

KAMITAN #1

I agree with you. Wasn't it people who built this city and all of the wonders of our modern technology.

KAMITAN #2

Yes, yes! People create other people too! We do not need the gods and goddesses for that!

(the two laugh)

KAMITAN #1

Ha, ha, ha. I know I certainly do not need any help in that area!

KAMITAN #2

Ha, ha, ha. I tell you. This conversation has helped me to make up my mind. I will no longer go to the temple. I am the master of my own life and I can do whatever I want. Who needs a feeble god anyway?

KAMITAN #1

I am with you, and when I meet with my other friends I will urge them to do the same.

(The two Egyptians exit and two others
enter. The first is pushing and shoving
the second. The second one falls to the
ground.)

KAMITAN #3
(from the ground)
Why have you resorted to violence in order to
resolve our differences? I will honor our agreement.

KAMITAN #4
(angrily)
I am tired of your promises. I want your land now!

KAMITAN #3

I told you that I cannot give it to you until the crop comes in. If that is not good enough let us go to the court of Ra and see what is fair. Let Ra tell us what is in accordance with Maat.

KAMITAN #4

What?! I do not care about any Maat! Ra is an old decrepit king. We now make out own rules. We have the right because we are the creators of this world and all good things in it.

KAMITAN #3
(incredulous-still on the ground)
What are you talking about? Ra created this world and all life.
KAMITAN #4
You believe in that nonsense? That is just a myth.
Ra told us that lie many years ago and now everyone believes it. Ra is nothing but a weak man and we owe him nothing. But you owe me land and I want it now!
Forget about Ra. Ra has grown old and he is powerless.

(Egyptian #4 pulls #3 up from the
ground and shoves him or her off stage.
the Scribe enters the stage on the left
side while Ra enters from the opposite
side of the stage in a pensive manner.)

SCRIBE
(passionate)

How can I say the things I must,
to record the story of the gods and goddesses is my trust.

But what I have seen in these times is clearly,
a most distressing sight in the eyes of the one who is ruling feebly.

Where is Maat in our land in these days?
The people have forgotten and follow unrighteous ways.

Where will the lust and the stealing end?
Can I dare to see another day of this trend?

Lo, I have seen what nobody should.
The ego of man going unchecked and misunderstood.

The land is full of foreigners and thieves and the lawless,
is there any wonder that our paradise is sinking into the deep and darkest abyss?

Besieged are we by the gangs and the robbers,
who pay off the unrighteous judges and lawyers.

Help us dear Lord in our time of need,
for we long to go back to the days of law and order and the righteous creed.

Hear me oh Ra and send down your law,
Maat is our only hope to reverse this evil flaw.

Send down your daughter, the fiery eye.
Let her destroy the unrighteous, thieves and tellers of the lie.

Let the waters of Maat cleanse our souls,
and bring us closer to the beauty of your holy abode.

(Ra seated at his throne)

RA

What is this that I have heard?
People say that I am old and decrepit and do not respect my word?

People have forgotten about me?
I who came up out of Nun in ancient times and created all from the elephant to the flea?

Into this world I brought Maat philosophy,
so that people could live in order and harmony.

What calamity has befallen the people!
What delusion or disease is this that causes them to utter such evil?

Ra pauses and walks a few steps around
the stage, thinking, then turns towards
the audience)

Goddess Worship and Rituals of Enlightenment

RA
(continuing)

How is it possible for people to have forgotten me and my power?
I created this world and it is I who sustain all life in it, even the most dainty flower.

If my eye were to close, the sun would cease to shine and all life would end!
What arrogance, What insolence, the people have been stricken with the diseases of greed, vanity, and conceit their mind does bend.

Like a good father I will visit upon them a punishment for this disrespect!
And this lesson they will surely never forget!

(Ra walks to the front of the stage,
facing audience and raises his arms and
calls out the following instructions.)

RA
(continuing)

Bring to me my Eye, I also call Nun and my children who were with me when I created creation.
Call the god Shu, the goddess Tefnut, the
god Geb and the goddess Nut to my attention.

(They enter from all directions and all run to the center of the stage and gather around Ra.)

RA
(continuing)

I have an important matter to discuss with you, who are my children.
I came into existence in primordial times and I created the universe and people, but now they are insulting me and treating me as those not from heaven.

They say I am old and feeble.
They do not keep the law which I have set down for all gods and people.

I feel like striking these evil ones down but I will wait to hear your valued opinion.
This decision I take not lightly for I know what will be its fruition.

Tell me my children, what do you think?
Should I take some action or should I turn and wink?

(Nu steps towards Ra)

NUN

Sire, the course you must follow is clear.
It is not right for people to insult you and forget the laws of righteousness and how they once regarded you as dear.

Furthermore, conceit, arrogance and selfishness lead to unhappiness and sorrow.

Show compassion and let your Eye go against these evil ones on the morrow.

Let it punish them utterly for their unrighteousness,
so that they may learn the lesson that humility is better than selfishness.

RA

Very well. Let my Eye come forth. Let my daughter
Hetheru come to me.

(The Eye is a female actress with the
symbol of the sun on her head. She
steps forward towards Ra and prostrates
at his feet.)

HETHERU

Here I am father.

RA

Dearest daughter, you are my fiery eye who shines on the entire world
and in the hearts of men and women.
You are the scorching power of the sun which sustains all of them.

However, there are evil men and women on the land.
They say I am old, and care not for my laws or the boons which I offer
with my own hand.

Go now to the world and seek out all the unrighteous people who are
speaking against me,
and kill them for their blasphemy.

Then, when this glorious duty I have given you is done,
come back to me and take your place at my side as the glorious flaming
power of the sun.

HETHERU

Oh radiant one who shines in my heart,
I will do as you say father, in this sacred duty I will play my part.

I will go to the world and I will seek out the evil ones and kill them
for your glory's sake,
to teach them you are still powerful and not weak, and to humble their
ego's mistake.

I will transform myself into the form of a lioness,
and I will roam the earth and destroy the evil men and women who are
lawless!

(They all walk off stage and then enter
Egyptian #1 and #2. They are still
talking against Ra)

KAMITAN #1

Ha, Ha, Ha, do you know a funny story I heard a while ago? A market
lady who was selling lettuce told me that Ra can hear everything and
see everything.

KAMITAN #2

Ha, ha, ha. What nonsense. What ignorance. What
fools believe in such things? We who are smart and strong do not
believe in such things.

(Egyptian #1 and Egyptian #2 start to
walk away but before they leave the
stage Hetheru comes in and her theme music is sung by the CHOIR.)

CHOIR

DUA HETHERU SEKHEMAAH...
DUA HETHERU SEKHEMAAH...
DUA HETHERU SEKHEMAAH...
DUA HETHERU SEKHEMAAH...

(the choir fades)
(See Note 1)

KAMITAN #2

Hey, what is that strange sound I hear?

HETHERU AS LIONESS
(roaring angrily)

Roarrrr...What is this I hear you have said about Ra?

KAMITAN #1
(turning around frightened)

Uh, uh nothing. We said nothing.

KAMITAN #2

Yes, yes we said nothing.

LIONESS

Do not lie to me! I heard all of your ridicule and pompous banter.

KAMITAN #1

Please, we did not mean anything.

KAMITAN #2

Who are you?

HETHERU AS LIONESS

I am Hetheru, the Eye of Ra and the avenger of Ra.

(The two Egyptians look at each other,
make a frightened expression and start
to back away in fear.)

HETHERU AS LIONESS
(continuing; sarcastically)

Where are you going? Did you not say that Ra is feeble and that you
control your own lives? Come now and show me your power.

(Egyptian #1 and #2 turn to go away and
get as far as the back of the stage but
Hetheru pounces on both of them there
and they remain down and unconscious.
Hetheru starts to bite at them and
after a minute gets off of them and
begins to lick her paws.)

HETHERU AS LIONESS
(continuing; to the audience)
Mmmmmm.....That was good! I could get to like this
job! I get to eat raw meat and people taste good! Mmmmmm.....

(Now enter KAMITANS #3 and #4 at the
front of the stage, not noticing
Hetheru and the two corpses. Egyptian
#4 is still shoving #3 and is now more
irate than before.)

KAMITAN #4
What is this you say? You still refuse me in my demands? I will teach
you a lesson on this day.

KAMITAN #3
(on his knees)
Please give me more time! Do not hurt me please!
Think of Ra and how he loves all people. Have mercy on me.

KAMITAN #4
(shoves #3 down on his back and pulls out a knife.)

The weak will be ruled by the strong. This is the way of things.
Do not speak of Ra who is weak and feeble.

(Egyptian #4 starts to kick #3. Then
Hetheru comes in the form of a lioness
and pounces on Egyptian #4 and pins him
down.)

HETHERU AS LIONESS
(roaring)
What is this I hear? You think that you are above the law? You say Ra
is feeble and weak? I am the power of Ra and I have come to deliver
his justice against all who speak and do evil in the world.

KAMITAN #4
(incredulous and frightened)
Please, please have mercy. I did not mean it! Have mercy on me!

HETHERU AS LIONESS
Your words come too late. Your sins are too many and your fate is
sealed.

(Hetheru bites at his neck and he dies.
Hetheru gets off of Egyptian #4 and

starts to lick her paws.)

KAMITAN #3
(happy, relieved)
Oh, thank you great one, you who have been sent by Ra. You have saved me. My faith is restored in the power and justice of the most high. The world has heard of your deeds and justice is returning to the land. Thank you.

(Egyptian #3 turns to leave the stage)

HETHERU AS LIONESS
(sarcastically)
And where do you think you are going? I am not finished with my meal yet.

(Realizing that she means to eat him
too Egyptian #3 turns to leave but
Hetheru lunges at him.)

KAMITAN #3
Please stop. Why are you threatening me? I have done no evil deeds?

HETHERU AS LIONESS
I no longer care for good or evil. All I want is flesh and blood of human bodies. From now on anyone who comes into my sight will be eaten at once. The more I eat, the more I want.

(The Egyptian gets away. She sits down
and licks her paws for a few minutes
and then turns to the audience.)

HETHERU AS LIONESS
(continuing)
What are you looking at? I am the power of the sun and now that I am in this form, my hunger is insatiable. I am addicted to flesh and blood and I am proud of it!

(Hetheru walks across the stage looking
at the audience in a stalking way and
then suddenly rushes down and pounces
on someone in the audience. Then she
returns to the stage and licks her paws
again.)

HETHERU AS LIONESS
(continuing)
Mmmmmm.... I love the taste of flesh and blood. I think I will stay here and eat to my heart's content. I like being the mistress of this world. It is sweet to my heart. I no longer care who is good or bad. I will eat them all!

KAMITAN #5 (O.S.)
Look out! Everybody run! There is the beast and she is coming our way!

HETHERU AS LIONESS
(sarcastically, turning to the sound that is coming from off stage)
Where can you hide, little people? I thought you were so powerful and proud? Come to me and show me how powerful you are.

(Hetheru runs off stage towards where
the sound came and then screams can be
heard.)

KAMITANS (O.S.)
Ahhhhh.... No, No,....Ahhhhh.... Roaring......
Screams.....More roaring and screams..29

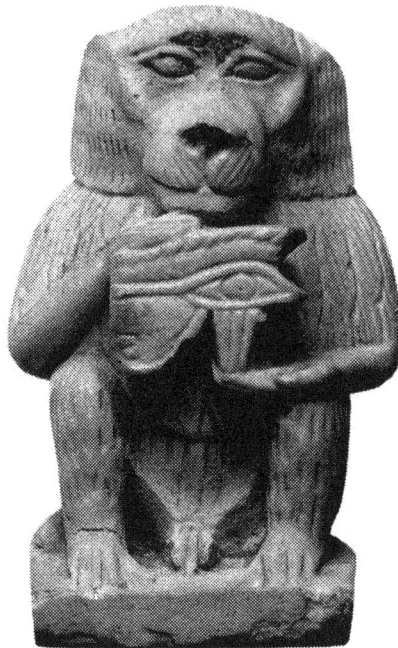

Above- actual statue of the god Djehuti holding the Divine Eye (Hetheru) which he heals through the wisdom teachings.

SCENE 2: THE DILEMMA

(Ra enters the stage.)

                              RA
                        (to himself)
I miss my beautiful daughter. Where is she? I sent her to do an important task for me and she has not yet returned.

(Ra calls out to Geb)

                              RA
                        (continuing)
Geb! Geb! Come here at once.

(Geb enters the stage and prostrates himself at the feet of Ra.)

                              RA
            (continuing; concerned, looking down with arms
                        folded behind him.)

What are these reports that I hear? Hetheru, my beautiful daughter, who shines brilliantly and who is the protector of my prestige on earth, has not returned?

                             GEB
                        (standing up)
I am afraid this is true, oh majestic one. Hetheru has taken to eating the flesh and blood of men and she has taken a great liking to it. And...

                              RA
                (looking up, intently on Geb.)
And what?

                             GEB
And, if she is not stopped soon she will destroy all men and women! You will have no more souls to revere you and to pay homage to you, great sire.

                              RA
So, the answer is clear. Go down and call her back. Bring her to me at once.

                             GEB
                        (timidly)
Well...

                              RA
                        (impatient)
Well, what? What is the problem now?

                             GEB
                    (bowing in shame)
I am sorry, father. No one is willing to go and look for her.

91

RA

Why not?

GEB

Because she is out of control.
She is devouring everything in her path and nobody, even the gods and
goddesses, can approach her or overcome her strength when she is on
patrol.

Such is her awesome strength and power,
that no one has the courage to face her thirst for violence at any
hour.

RA

What do you mean?
She is my precious daughter, the light of the universe and the most
beautiful goddess in existence and the most wonderful queen.

GEB

Yes my lord, but she has become deluded with power
and the lust of flesh and blood!

RA
(surprised)

What is this you say!
How is it possible for the lady of love, the light of the shining sun,
the goddess of beauty herself, to fall into the dream of mortal
existence for even one day?

GEB

I do not know, exalted one. I do not know.

RA

If all of you are too afraid of her and she is too powerful to
overcome,
then we must use cunning in order to stop her and guile to reverse the
deluded character she has become.

GEB

Sire, how will we do this dangerous and heroic deed?

RA

Send messengers to the city of Abu and have mandrakes brought to me
here.
Then have the maidservants bruise the grain for making beer.

Let them make it in great quantities.
This takes precedence above all priorities.

Then call upon my minister, Lord Djehuti
and have him report to me at once because I will charge him with an
important duty!

GEB

Yes my Lord at once.
(Geb exits stage. Ra sits on a throne
and waits.)

SCENE 3: THE PLAN TO SAVE HETHERU

RA

(with a heavy heart)

What will become of my daughter, Hetheru, the light of the sun, my very eye?
What will become of the people of the earth, who are my very own creations, part of my very soul if they cannot hide?

(Geb returns with two servants. They
are carrying jugs and baskets.)

GEB

I have returned sire, with the items you requested with mandrakes from the city of Abu,
and beer from our own city of Anu.

RA

Now call my son, the minister of all my affairs,
Lord Djehuti at once.

GEB

He is on his way here at this very moment beloved
Grandsire.

(Enter Djehuti. He walks up to the
throne and prostrates himself at the
feet of Ra.)

DJEHUTI AS IBIS

Oh majestic one, Creator of the universe and exalted spirit of spirits.
Oh glorious one, foremost in the great boat of creation and sire of the gods and goddesses.
How may I serve you on this day?

Goddess Worship and Rituals of Enlightenment

RA

Oh great one of words and enlightener of hearts, a great calamity has befallen my daughter.
The lady of beauty and light is lost in the world as a raging beast without a halter.

She has forgotten me and her exalted position among the stars.
She is bent on destroying humanity and will soon leave it desolate if she continues as she has so far.

Now that she is gone from the heavens, the universe has no defense.
The forces of darkness and evil are encroaching upon the universe because she no longer forces them into silence.

A great calamity this is indeed!

DJEHUTI AS IBIS
(concerned)
What can I do to help, oh majestic one?

RA

She has taken the form of a lioness and she is out of control, rampaging all over the world seeking victims whom unrighteousness they have sold their soul.
You must bring her back to me.
You of all the gods and goddesses are the most cunning and well spoken in-deed.

Only you can gain her confidence and convince her to return to her rightful place.
This sacred task is a danger which I ask you to face.

DJEHUTI AS IBIS

Well spoken I am indeed my Lord,
but how will I speak to her if she will devour anyone before they have a chance to say a foreword?

RA

We have created a special potion of mandrake and beer.
We will mix it with the blood that she likes to drink so much and you will have a chance to reach her ear.

This will cause her to fall into a deep sleep.
Then you can surely approach her, since in this state she will be sluggish and weak.

DJEHUTI AS IBIS

A good plan indeed this is but there is something more that is necessary.

RA

What else?

DJEHUTI AS IBIS

If she sees me in this form when she wakes up she will surely believe that I am a threat to her.
So I must distract her until I am able to gain her confidence and trust and the delusion of her mind be the conqueror.

RA

What will you do?

DJEHUTI AS IBIS

I will transform my self into the form of a lowly baboon,
and surely I will appear harmless and meek when she comes out of her
swoon.

RA

Ahhh... Well said, I approve of this plan.
Go now and bring her back to me safely to my loving hand.

For the fate of men and women and the universe hangs in the balance,
and the life of the lady of light too is in danger from this evil
trance!

DJEHUTI AS IBIS
(with upraised arms)
I will leave at once my Lord.

RA

Hetepu! Peace be with you.

(Hetheru appears in the center of the
stage, licking her paws. Off stage
moans and groans from her victims can
be heard.)

VICTIMS
Uhh.........hh.........Uhh.........Uhh........
Somebody please help us....Uhh........ Ahh........

HETHERU AS LIONESS
(arrogantly, callously)
Oh be silent! Nobody can help you now. You are here to serve me and I
can do whatever I want. There is no power above mine and I will enjoy
all the pleasures of the earth according to my will and desire.

(more groans can be heard and then a
noise in the opposite direction. Two
Egyptians have placed the jugs on the
stage and quickly run away. Hetheru now
notices some jugs and moves towards
them fearlessly.)

HETHERU AS LIONESS
(continuing)
Who is there? Do you dare to approach me, the mistress of this land? I
will devour you for daring to commit such an outrage!

(Noticing the jugs she puts a paw into
it and then puts it to her mouth.)

HETHERU AS LIONESS
(continuing)
Mmmm...... Blood wine! Just the way I like it.

(She picks up one jug and then drinks
the whole thing. Then she picks up the
other jug and does the same.)

HETHERU AS LIONESS
(continuing; laying down, rubbing her stomach)
That was nice. I think I will now enjoy some sleep.
Yes...Eat, drink and sleep, there is nothing better to do in the
world. Mmmm........

(She finds a comfortable spot in the
center of the stage and then lays her
head down to sleep. Djehuti approaches
her stealthily. He is now in his baboon
form.)

DJEHUTI AS BABOON
(whispering, with upraised arms)

Look at the beautiful daughter of Ra.
Such degradation you have come to, from beauty to beast, from smile to
a grimace, from compassionate goddess to animal you have come very
far.

Once you were the life of the court of Ra, the very radiance of the
universe itself,
and what has become of you now as you lay there not knowing your true
inner self?

I promise you that I will make every effort to help you,
to cure this delusion which has taken hold and distorted what is true.

I promise to help you and to bring you back to take your rightful
place,
as the most exalted of gods and goddesses, the worlds above and below
ever to grace.

I will help you to remember your glory of the past,
and the wonders which you have forgotten, his is my task.

(He crept closer to her and made
noise to announce his approach.
When Hetheru woke and realized that
something was approaching she
immediately took an offensive stance
and prepared to fight. Then Djehuti
called out:)

Goddess Worship and Rituals of Enlightenment

DJEHUTI AS BABOON
(continuing)
Hail O beautiful daughter of the Sun!
(As soon as Hetheru notices that it is
only a baboon she takes poise and
immediately Djehuti asks if he could
speak with her.)

DJEHUTI AS BABOON
(continuing)
Exalted mistress of the world, may I approach to speak with you?

HETHERU AS LIONESS
Say what you have to say and then I will eat you!

DJEHUTI AS BABOON
You certainly have the power to kill me,
but you should think about the "parable of the vulture and the
wildcat" which I will tell thee.

If you kill me you will never find out about it.
And this would be a great loss for you since there is so much food in
the sage's writ.

HETHERU AS LIONESS
(growling-raising voice)
What is this parable? Tell me right now I desire to know this instant!

(Then she sits down. Djehuti began to
speak immediately so as to keep her
attention captivated with interest.)

DJEHUTI AS BABOON
(cautiously)
There was a mother vulture and a mother wildcat who were close
neighbors.
The vulture had four chicks and the wildcat had
given birth to four kittens but though they were
living close by they never did each other any
favors.

The mother vulture and the mother wildcat had a big problem.
If either left the area they feared that the children, the other
mother would harm them.

Their children were hungry but the two mothers were both afraid,
to leave them alone because they feared that either one of them would
kill the other's children for food so there they stayed.

The two mothers arranged a truce between them by upon the name of Ra
an oath swearing.
They swore that neither one would hurt the other's children and then
in peace to go for food hunting.

So now they both felt secure enough to go out and start hunting food
for their children.

For some time the truce worked and soon the vulture chicks and the kittens began to grow and fend.

One day one of the vulture chicks went to the area where the kittens were playing and he snatched away a portion of their food.
One of the kittens reached out and swatted the chick and injured it and told it to find its own edibles, he was so rude.

The chick could not fly because of the injury, but had enough strength to tell the kitten,
"you have broken the oath between our families and
Ra will punish you for this great injustice that to me you have given."

When the mother vulture returned she noticed that her chick was lying on the ground, dead, so she figured that the wildcat had broken her promise.
The next time that the wildcat left to go hunting the mother vulture killed all of the kittens and brought them back to her nest for food thinking there was no witness.

When the mother wildcat returned she realized that the mother vulture had killed her kittens.
So she cried out to Ra, "O Divine one, you who uphold righteousness, punish the evil doer who has broken the oath which was sworn upon your name, the "Lord of Justice," which Maat has written!

Ra heard this plea and set the plan in motion,
to carry out the punishment for this horrible transgression.

The next day as the mother vulture was hunting she came upon a campfire which had a portion of meat being cooked and there was no one in sight to make
intervention.
She swooped down and grabbed it and quickly returned to her nest with the intention,

to drop it in her nest for her chicks to feast on, and take care of their hunger and be a good mother thereupon.

But she had not noticed that there was a smoldering piece of coal attached to the meat.
The nest caught fire and the three chicks were burnt to death because she could not set foot in the nest, so hot was it to her feet.

Noticing this the mother wildcat yelled out, "You killed my children and now Ra has punished you because of this unrighteous bout!"

(Djehuti pauses for a moment. Hetheru
has stopped licking herself and is
silent. Then she speaks.)

Goddess Worship and Rituals of Enlightenment

HETHERU AS LIONESS

Is this a true story? Does Ra really care for such an insignificant creature? Does he have such power to give justice even to a wildcat?

DJEHUTI AS BABOON

Oh glorious lady, do you see,
the omniscience and justice of Ra, who sees and hears all things that cannot we?

He is the giver of life and all of nature owes its existence to him.
He controls every particle of Creation and can end all Creation with a single whim.

He is the sustainer of Creation and His justice is perfect.
Praises be to him and praises be to you who are his daughter in effect!

(Hetheru began to reflect upon the
meaning of this parable and she
began to remember her father and the
wonderful relationship they shared in
the past.)

HETHERU AS LIONESS
(looking down in a pensive manner)
What you say about Ra sounds familiar to me somehow ...but I don't know...

(Djehuti took advantage of the
opportunity and moved closer to her and
said)

DJEHUTI AS BABOON

Oh Heavenly lady, I bring you an offering of divine food from the abode of the Sun God Ra.
It brings health and joy to all who eat it as well as peace to your spirit, your Ka.

(Hetheru began to relax and saw no harm
in accepting the tribute from the
humble baboon.)
(As the beautiful goddess consumes the
offering Djehuti begins to speak again).

DJEHUTI AS BABOON
(continuing)
These herbs come from the land of Kamit, where we were born, the beautiful Ta-mery.
Kamit is the first land which rose up from Nun, the Primeval Waters, in ancient times of history.

It was created for the gods and goddesses and the righteous people, all children of Ra.
It is also the home of your Divine Father and your brother Shu but now they all seem so far.

All beings long to return to the land of their birth.
Who can be happy living away from the very source of happiness and
live in such hunger and thirst?

(Hetheru had forgotten her true
identity and became addicted to the
taste of blood. But now she begins to
remember the wonder of her Divine
Father, Kamit and her own true
identity. She began to think about her
temples in Kamit and how men and women
had brought her offerings and revered
her beauty as the most exalted of
all goddesses. Hetheru was
overwhelmed by these memories and
feelings that she began to cry.)

HETHERU AS LIONESS
(sobbing)
Can this be true? Am I in reality the beautiful goddess of light? How
could I have left such glory and fallen to such degradation?

DJEHUTI AS BABOON
(coming closer to her with sincerity)
Oh Great Lady, you are crying now but think of the pain of the people
in Kamit who are deprived of your glories.
Due to your absence there is no merriment, no singing, no parties in
Kamit and the demons of chaos are going unpunished, bringing to Ra
untold worries.

Return with me and I will tell you more stories of
Kamit.
These will enlighten you as I relate the sagas and tales of happiness
and regret.

(As soon as she heard this, Hetheru
realizes that he is trying to get her
to go back to Kamit and she becomes
exceedingly angry. She roars and made
terrible sounds and Djehuti
immediately prostrates himself and begs
for mercy in the name of Ra)

HETHERU AS LIONESS
(flaring with anger over him)
Rrrrrrrrrr!

DJEHUTI AS BABOON
Wait! Wait just one minute!

(Short pause as Hetheru pulls herself
together and begins to realize what
Djehuti is trying to do)

HETHERU AS LIONESS
(continuing)

What is this? You are trying to trick me! You want me to leave this place where I am the absolute monarch and where I can act on all of my desires at will? You want me to go back to Kamit and give all of this up? I will eat you right now for your treachery!

DJEHUTI AS BABOON
(prostrating and acting as if in fear)

Oh Divine Lady before you kill me listen to this important parable about the two vultures.

HETHERU AS LIONESS
(calming down from the rage)

What? What? Tell me quickly, and then I will kill you.

(Hetheru calmed down because she was intrigued by the words of Djehuti. She sat down again and started to lick her paws. He quickly began to speak.)

DJEHUTI AS BABOON

Once upon a time there were two vultures in the forest. One said to the other, "My eyes are so perfect that I can see all things to the end of the earth and beyond that also the rest."

The other vulture said "Well I can hear everything." "I can even hear Ra as he decrees the fate of all Creation and of every being."

The two vultures debated about which gift is better. The vulture with the keen hearing said, "another bird far away told me that an insect was eaten by a lizard who was more clever.

The lizard was then eaten by a snake and then the snake was caught by a hawk. The snake was so heavy that the snake and the hawk fell into the sea as they fought.

The vulture with keen hearing asked, "Can you tell me what is happening now by looking with your keen eyesight?" The vulture with the keen eyesight replied, "the falcon and the snake have been swallowed by a fish and that fish was swallowed up by a larger fish of greater might.

The bigger fish came to close to shore and a lion grabbed it out of the sea. Then a legendary creature called griffin flew to the area and carried off the lion as easy as plucking a weed.

One vulture said to the other, "this remarkable scene that we have witnessed proves the power of Ra. Even the existence of the fly was noticed and the consequence of killing will be punished by one's own death no matter how near or far.

But how is it that the griffin has survived all of this while the other animals who committed violence reaped the reward for their actions?"
The other vulture answered, "It must be that the griffin is the messenger of Ra who was sent to carry out the law of Ra's retributions.

The griffin is the most powerful of all creatures.
It is God's own ultimate instrument of right and truth which enforces the law in all the world's quarters."

HETHERU AS LIONESS
(curiously)
Is there really such a creature that is more powerful than any other, even me? Is Ra's perfection so complete as to provide for every creature in this universe? How is this possible?

(Djehuti begins to explain the moral of
the parable.)

DJEHUTI AS BABOON
Oh Great Lady, do you see how the Divine Father rewards goodness with goodness and evil with punishment?
In this manner the balance of the universe is maintained by the Great God in all his glory and to the world's last filament.

Oh great lady, you have been endowed with Ra's power.
You are the Eye of Ra in it's greatest hour.

You have the power to carry out the law of the universe.
It is YOU who are the most powerful force in all of Creation, indeed of all beings you are foremost, you come first.

(After hearing this the goddess's eyes
filled with joy and she began to feel
pride in being the daughter of Ra. She
told Djehuti)

HETHERU AS LIONESS
You may now relax, humble one. I no longer desire to kill and eat you. Your words have captivated me and I know now that you are a beneficent being.
Something in me has stirred, but I do not yet know what it is fully.

DJEHUTI AS BABOON
Very good my lady, the memory of your deeper self is returning.
Let us walk towards the land of Kamit and as we do
I shall tell you more wonders and glories of Kamit and Ra, about you and the truth you are seeking.

HETHERU AS LIONESS
Very well, but first tell me, who are you and how is it that you know these parables and mysteries?

DJEHUTI AS BABOON
(smiling)
All in good time my dear, all in good time.

Soon you will have the answers to all of your questions and the way of the quest your are on soon you will find.

For now listen and things will become clear very soon.
For as the mind becomes clear through wisdom you will make sense of the thoughts that in your mind loom.

(They began to walk towards Kamit -back and forth across the stage- and Djehuti begins to recite another parable.)

DJEHUTI AS BABOON
(continuing)

Once upon a time there were two jackals who were to each other a friend.
One day, as they rested, suddenly they saw a lion running towards them with intentions for them to rend.

Much to the lion's surprise they did not attempt to run away.
When the lion reached them it stopped and asked them why they acted in this way?

The jackals replied that the lion would catch them anyway so there was no point in running away and getting tired in a futile effort to escape.
The lion was so pleased with their calm and truthful answer that he spared their life and let them go on their way with all haste.

HETHERU AS LIONESS

Ha ha ha! That one was truly amusing. Ha ha ha! You are a truly good storyteller. Your parables have such true meaning and they are reflecting the way I feel at this moment. I spared your life because I too see honesty in you and a calmness that I cannot describe. Please tell me more, for I am enjoying these teachings.

DJEHUTI AS BABOON
(smiling)

I am pleased that you are pleased my lady.
Let us walk further towards Kamit and I will protect you on the way to Ta-mery."

(Hetheru, raised her eyebrow at him as soon as she heard this and replied- becoming a little cocky, having learned a little knowledge)

HETHERU AS LIONESS
(sarcastically-humorously)

How can you protect me? The Eye of the Sun is the most powerful force and it needs no protection, especially from a baboon!

DJEHUTI AS BABOON
The strong sometimes need help from those who are weaker.
Do you know the parable of the mouse and the lion, it is truly a pleaser?

I will tell you and you will understand.
For knowing this teaching brings the glory of God closer at hand.

(Djehuti began to tell the parable as
they walked towards Kamit again)

DJEHUTI AS BABOON
Long ago there was a lion who lived as a king in the forest.
He was so powerful that all the other animals feared him more than all the rest.

One day the lion came upon a panther who was badly wounded.
The lion asked the panther who had injured him and the panther told him that man was responsible for all his injuries included.

The lion never heard of a creature called "man" and he decided to hunt this creature and punish him with the lion's own hand.

On the way to find man the lion met a mule, an ox, a cow, a bear and another lion which had all by man been captured.
All of them had been outsmarted by man even though they were more powerful and by their parents well- tutored.

They all said that man was the most cunning creature,
In all of the forest there was no equal to his viciousness as a feature.

Even though man appeared to be feeble and weak.
They told the powerful lion to stay away from man so as to live beyond this very week.

This only made the lion more determined to find man.
On the way the lion came across a small mouse and wanted to swat it dead with his paw like a fan.

Without a thought the lion raised a paw to crush the mouse but the mouse pleaded for mercy and pledged to be the lion's friend in the time of need.
The lion asked him, "How can you ever help me, I am more powerful than any creature indeed."

The mouse replied, "Do not be so arrogant and sure of yourself.
Sometimes the weak can help the powerful, to safeguard their very health."

For his own amusement the lion let the mouse go and went on his way.
Soon after that encounter with the mouse the lion fell into a pit and was tangled up in a net so strongly that he could not escape man's cold-hearted play.

The lion expected to die the next day when man would find him.
But suddenly, the lion heard a screeching little voice coming from a nearby tree limb.

It was the little mouse who had returned true to his word.
And here began the legend that was never before heard.

The mouse worked upon the ropes all night,
and before man could come to check the net with the morning's light,
the lion had been freed from the terrible death trap.
The enduring gratitude of the lion for getting him out of the serious mishap.

So great lady, remember that every power will someday meet a higher power and the weak can sometimes help those who are strong,
to escape from the tough situations when they find themselves in a tight wrap and they are forced to sing a depressing song.

HETHERU AS LIONESS
Mmmm..... Your parable is intriguing but I don't know. I will still rely on my own strength rather than on the friendship of a mouse.

(Before entering the city of Waset
(Thebes) Hetheru laid down to rest)

DJEHUTI AS BABOON
Great lady, we have reached the outer boundary of the city of Waset.
Let us rest here and then go into the city tomorrow after some needed rest.

HETHERU AS LIONESS
Very well. I have grown tired from the journey and I feel a strange slumber coming over me. Before I sleep I wish to tell you of my gratitude. I want to thank you for awakening in me some feelings and memories which I had forgotten. Looking at things now it seems that I was lost even when I thought I was happy where I was. You are the best of teachers and I salute you.

(Hetheru bows her head and raises her
harms to Djehuti as a gesture of
respect)

DJEHUTI AS BABOON
Thank you my lady, I am always your humble servant.
Sleep now and be free of worry for I am here to watch over you as the situation may warrant.

HETHERU AS LIONESS
(sarcastically, humorously-acknowledging his
wisdom but not his physical capacity)

Yeaaaa right.

DIM LIGHTS

(Hetheru lays down to sleep. Djehuti, ignoring her last remark, sits in the cross-legged position, facing the audience but looking around every few seconds. On the far right side of the stage there are two characters wearing serpent costumes talking. The enemies of Ra were not pleased with her return so they plotted against her. In the middle of the night they sent a serpent of chaos to poison her in order to leave Ra defenseless, deprived of his protecting Eye.)

DEMON #1
We are the demons of the earth and we have the right to rule over this earth.

DEMON #2
Yes! If Djehuti succeeds in bringing Hetheru back to Kamit we will be destroyed.

DEMON #1
It is time. Release the serpent that will strike her down and leave Ra without the power of his Eye, the radiance of the sun which pours out light on all.
Let everything fall into darkness and chaos.

(The demons released the serpent but Djehuti, who was vigilant all of the time, noticed the serpent and woke Hetheru.)

DJEHUTI AS BABOON
Hetheru, awaken immediately, there is a danger before us!

HETHERU AS LIONESS
What is it? Where is this danger?

DJEHUTI AS BABOON
(jumping up and down and pointing towards the serpent)
Look behind you, an evil serpent approaches!

(Still in the form of a lioness, Hetheru leaps on the serpent and broke the serpent's back.)

Goddess Worship and Rituals of Enlightenment

DJEHUTI AS BABOON
(continuing)
Look over there, those two released the serpent.
They are demons, enemies of your father Ra. You must stop them also.

(The demons try to leave but Hetheru
runs after them off stage and then back
on stage. She pounces on them but does
not kill them.)

HETHERU AS LIONESS
Lord Djehuti what should I do with them now? I have lost the appetite
for killing, meat eating and the drinking of blood.

DJEHUTI AS BABOON
Very good my lady, you have lost the desire for violence and have
turned towards righteousness.
Very good, very good, I see in you the glowing light heavenliness.

Tie them up and Ra will punish them in accordance with their crimes.
You have performed your duty well, and thus, your enlightenment is at
hand for I have seen all the signs.

(After tying them up Hetheru walks over
to Djehuti.)

HETHERU AS LIONESS
Dear master, you have saved my life today. I now see the wisdom of
your parable of the lion and the mouse. I am that lion and you are the
humble mouse who has saved me.

DJEHUTI AS BABOON
(smiling)
I am pleased that you have placed your confidence in me.
It is this same confidence that will completely liberate you from your
bondage to the animal passion you now experience and can now clearly
see.

HETHERU AS LIONESS
What do you mean teacher? Am I not liberated already? You said
yourself that I have tuned away from violence and desire. What more is
there?

DJEHUTI AS BABOON
You have turned toward what is righteous and good but this is only the
beginning.
Now you must realize your true nature and take your true form as it
was when Ra created the first morning.

HETHERU AS LIONESS
But how can I do that, I feel lost. And the thought of losing this
body, that I have grown so used to, causes fear in my heart! I do not
know what to do next. Please direct me great sir. Teacher to my heart,
show me the way for I feel lost.

DJEHUTI AS BABOON
Have no fear; this is the time of greatest importance,
because you are letting go of your ignorance.

The ignorance of the past melts away as you are discovering your true nature.
I will lead you through the murky waters of ignorance into the light of the day of understanding and liberated pleasure.

Just as a lotus rises through the muddy water,
I will show you the way to the light which is the greatest awakener.

HETHERU AS LIONESS
(reassured)
Dear teacher, your words are reassuring to the heart. Please tell me, what should I do in order to be completely free from my delusion?

DJEHUTI AS BABOON
Now is the time that you must remember yourself fully.
Sit beside me and close your eyes and place your trust in me completely.

(They both sit in cross-legged position
at the front of the stage-facing
audience.)

DJEHUTI AS BABOON
(continuing)
Now repeat after me:
DUA **RA**, DUA **RA**, DUA **RA**, KHEPHERA

HETHERU AS LIONESS
DUA **RA**, DUA **RA**, DUA **RA**, KHEPHERAAAA.....
DJEHUTI AS BABOON
DUA **RA**, DUA **RA**, DUA **RA**, KHEPHERA.....

HETHERU AS LIONESS
DUA **RA**, DUA **RA**, DUA **RA**, KHEPHERA...

CHOIR
(softly as Djehuti and Hetheru speak and then
fading to silence)
DUA **RA**, DUA **RA**, DUA **RA**, KHEPHERA...
DUA **RA**, DUA **RA**, DUA **RA**, KHEPHERA...
DUA **RA**, DUA **RA**, DUA **RA**, KHEPHERA...
(See Note 2)

DJEHUTI AS BABOON
Now close your eyes, relax and breath in deeply.
As you become more calm and feel a lightness in your body.
Now feel the warmth that is in your heart, the warmth of peace and divine glory.

HETHERU AS LIONESS
I feel it. I feel it.

DJEHUTI AS BABOON
Very well. Now go deeper and deeper. Look for the light within your heart.

HETHERU AS LIONESS
(exited)

I see it! I see it!

DJEHUTI AS BABOON

Now feel the radiance and purity of the light, the
goodness and love within the light..

HETHERU AS LIONESS
(swooning)

Ahh......

DJEHUTI AS BABOON

Very good. Now relax and allow the light to fill your mind.
Give yourself completely to the light of your own heart and don't hold
back, cross into infinity, step over the line.

HETHERU AS LIONESS

I see someone in the light.

DJEHUTI AS BABOON

Who do you see?

HETHERU AS LIONESS

It is a woman. I cannot see her face but she seems familiar. She is
beautiful and strong, virtuous and merciful.

DJEHUTI AS BABOON

Where is she?

HETHERU AS LIONESS

She is in a great palace.

DJEHUTI AS BABOON

What is she doing?

HETHERU AS LIONESS

She is talking to a man who is seated at the throne.
She is worshipping him and now he is blessing her.

DJEHUTI AS BABOON

Go over to her and look at her face.

HETHERU AS LIONESS
(surprised)

Uhh...

DJEHUTI AS BABOON

What do you see?

HETHERU AS LIONESS

It is me! It is me! I am that great lady in the palace of Anu. I am the daughter of the mighty God Ra. I am that Griffin. I was lost as the vicious lioness and now I have found my way!

DJEHUTI AS BABOON
(voice rising gradually, urging and insistent)

Now rise up my child and assume your true form and leave this degraded lioness body for all time.
Be free from the desire for violence, flesh and blood and take your place among the gods and goddesses which your true place to find.
Rise up my child, rise up and remember your true nature!
Come now and discover the joy of being God's
pleasure.

CHOIR
(softly as Djehuti and Hetheru speak and then
fading to silence)

Hetheru aha, m Sekhem aah ten Neteritaa
(Hetheru, raise yourself up in your true form as the great goddess of Power (Life Force))

Ten Nebetawi, Ten Neberdjer, Uben tawi
(You are the mistress of the world, you are all encompassing divinity, the light of the world)

Rekhit iri, neteru iri, anetj k ren
(The people on earth and the gods and goddesses all praise your name)

Ten Nebetawi, Ten Neberdjer, ten Neterit aah nefert
(You are the mistress of the world, you are all encompassing divinity, the great goddess of beauty.) (see Note 3)

(They both stand up and raise their
arms. Hetheru takes off the costume and
steps out of it gracefully. LIGHTS ON
Hetheru)

DJEHUTI AS BABOON
(continuing)

Ahhhhh... That's better, much better. Dua Hetheru!
Dua Hetheru! Hail to you great lady of fire and light!

(Djehuti parades her around the stage
once.)

HETHERU AS WOMAN
(joyous)

I am Hetheru! I am Hetheru!

DJEHUTI AS BABOON

Now we are ready to enter into the city.
You will not believe how happy the people will be to see you, they are
more than ready.

(They walk off the stage and then enter
some KAMITANs, holding flowers.)

KAMITAN #6

Have you heard the great news?

KAMITAN #7

Yes and I am excited beyond measure. Hetheru is returning to us. Our
lady of light is returning to us!

(Hetheru and Djehuti walk in and all
the people prostrate themselves in
front of Hetheru.)

HETHERU AS WOMAN

Thank you all for your praises and support.
I was lost in the wilderness of life but now I have found my way again
to Ra's divine court.
I pledge to take care of you, as I always have, and to love you with
all of my heart as the goddess of love, beauty and glory of all sorts.

CROWD
                                    (cheering)
Dua Hetheru! Dua Hetheru! Dua Hetheru!
Dua Hetheru! Dua Hetheru!...

DJEHUTI AS BABOON

Look dear one, the entire city is rejoicing at your return!

CROWD
                        (cheering)
Dua Hetheru!Dua Hetheru!Dua Hetheru!Dua Hetheru! DuaHetheru!

DJEHUTI AS BABOON

Now dearest, it is time that you see me in my true
form.

(Hetheru steps back as Djehuti takes
off his costume, revealing himself as
a man with the head of an Ibis bird-his
true form.)

HETHERU AS WOMAN

It is, it is you! Lord Djehuti!

(Hetheru prostrates herself at
Djehuti's feet.)

HETHERU AS WOMAN
(continuing)

Dear Uncle, I knew it was you.
Somehow I felt you in your words, so true.

A greater teacher I could not have had.
Adorations to you a thousand times, Oh Lord today I am more than glad!

(As Djehuti bends over, grabs her
shoulder and lifts her up, enter Ra,
Geb and the other gods and goddesses.
On seeing Ra, Hetheru runs to him and
prostrates herself and then hugs him.)

RA
(smiling)

Oh dearest daughter, I always knew you would come back to me.
The skilful words of Lord Djehuti have once again brightened the light
which had gone dim and nobody else could see.

From this time on I decree that the baboon form which Djehuti used
shall be revered for all time as a sign of wisdom and truth-speaking.
I further proclaim that the lioness form will forever be remembered as
the symbol of strength and power for all time, with ancient traditions
in keeping.

From this day forth, future generations will celebrate the return of
my daughter.
Festivals of joy and laughter will fill the air and this homecoming
will never be forgotten forever.

This story will enlighten hearts and they will be freed;
anyone who listens to it from the slavery of evil in thought, word or
deed.

I am Ra and my word is Maat, that which is true.
Those who follow the wise will be led to discover what know only the
few.

Therefore, a life of righteousness will praise my light which is in
the heart of all creatures,
watching over all who's desire for enlightenment this story will be
their teacher.

(All the players come from stage right
in a procession.
The first four are carrying a palanquin
on which sits a box that is covered
with a cloth. The next three players
are playing drum, tambourine and
sistrum (male on drums-females on
tambourine and sistrum). The procession
walks along the back of the stage to
the opposite side and then turns
towards the front and then, after
reaching the front of the stage, turn
towards the center. The players
carrying the palanquin set it down at

the front-center of the stage. Ra
unveils the cloth and a statue of
Hetheru becomes visible.)

CHOIR
(with amazement)

Aaahhhh...

(After a few moments uuing and ahhing
the group in procession begin the
following chant.)

CHOIR
(continuing)

Ommmm! Ommmm! Ommmm! Ommmm!
Hetheru gem wat, Hetheru gem wat!

Hetheru has found her way,
into our hearts and to the day.
Forever more the light she brings,
is life eternal and endless spring.

CHOIR
(continuing)

Dua Hetheru! Neterit Aah! (see Note 4)
Dua Hetheru! Neterit Aah!
Dua Hetheru! Sekhem Aah! Dua Hetheru! Sekhem Aah!
Dua Hetheru! NebeTawi! Dua Hetheru! NebeTawi!
Dua Hetheru!.... Dua Hetheru!....

Adorations to Hetheru, the great goddess.
Adorations to Hetheru, the great power.
Adorations to Hetheru, the mistress of the earth.
Adorations to Hetheru, Adorations to Hetheru...

(Lights on statue and the players close
to it. Djehuti begins to pour a
libation in front of the statue.
Hetheru brings burning incense and
places it in front of the statue. Ra
places a lit candle in front of the
statue.)

CHOIR
(continuing)

Hah! Hetheru Ra Djehuti,
Hah! Hetheru Ra Djehuti...
Hah! Hetheru Ra Djehuti,
Hah! Hetheru Ra Djehuti...
Hail Hetheru, Ra and Djehuti,
Hail Hetheru, Ra and Djehuti!...

(The players break out of the choir and
begin to dance around the stage in
various directions, not wildly but not
structured and also not inhibited.
Different players utter the following
words at the same time but not
synchronized. The drumming and
tambourine rise in intensity, volume
and rhythm)

CROWD

Hetheru Sheta,
Hetheru Sheta,
Shemsu Hetheru,
Mery mut Hetheru!
Mery mut Hetheru!

The mysteries of Hetheru, we follow those. Hetheru is our beloved
mother!

Neru Hetheru Akhu! Akhu!
Neru Hetheru Akhu! Akhu!

Victory of Hetheru Glory! Glory!
Victory of Hetheru Glory! Glory!
Glory! Glory! Glory! Glory!...

Neru Hetheru Akhu! Akhu!
Neru Hetheru Akhu! Akhu!
Neru Hetheru Akhu! Akhu!
Neru Hetheru Akhu! Akhu!...

(As the chanting goes on, Ra, Hetheru,
Djehuti exit stage left. Picking up the
palanquin, the rest of the players all
Exit stage as chanting goes on and
fades as the curtain comes down.)

(THE END)

Notes on the music for the play.

1. This recording is available on the CD *Adorations to Ra and Hetheru* by Muata Ashby. *Dua Hetheru Neterit-aah* means Adorations to Hathor, the great goddess of Life Force Power. In Ancient Egyptian the term *Sekhem* means Life Force energy, like the Chi of the Chinese and Prana of the Indian Yoga mystics. In her aspect as Sekhmet, Hetheru displays her power in much the same way as the goddess Durga displays her power in her aspect as of Kali. This song was performed in the Phrygian mode. It is ***Lively, exciting and devotional***. Instruments used: Vocal, Nefer, Sistrum, Cymbals, Tar, Drone Choir. It has a driving beat that extols the energy of the goddess. Instruments used: Vocal, Nefer, Sistrum, Cymbals, Tar, Drone Choir.

2. This recording is available on the CD *Adorations to Ra and Hetheru* by Muata Ashby. *Dua Ra Khepera* means Adorations to Ra in the form of Khepera. These words of power are based on the mythology related to the Supreme Being who manifests in the Ra-Khepera, the Creator, the form of the morning sun which creates the day or brings it into being with his rising. Its attitude is lively, exciting and devotional, designed for late morning listening. Instruments used: Vocals, Nefer, Sistrum, Clapping, and Tar.

3. This song was a continuation of the devotional music to the goddess which began in my second CD, Adorations to Ra and Hetheru). Its melody and the use of ancient and modern musical instruments bring the feeling of the goddess alive for our times. It is a joy to sing and an honor to be given the opportunity to be used as her voice. This song was inspired also by the famous festivals of Hetheru, which were the most popular festive occasions in Ancient Egyptian culture. Therefore, it is lively and suitable for singing along as well as dancing. This recording is available on the CD *Haari Om* by Muata Ashby.

4. This recording is available on the CD *Adorations to Ra and Hetheru* by Muata Ashby. *Dua Hetheru Neterit-aah* means Adorations to Hathor, the great goddess. It was written in the Dorian Mode. It is a devotional to the goddess in her form as the great mistress of the universe. It was written in an expansive mood, feeling the glory of the Divine and the warmth of the feminine aspect of the Divine. The long commencement of the song with the sistrum is a homage to the goddess as it is her special musical instrument, used to awaken the *Arat* serpent power (known as Kundalini) in Indian mysticism. Instruments used: Vocal, Nefer, Sistrum, Tar, Drone Choir. *Dua Hetheru Neterit-aah* is the first line in a poem written by Muata Ashby based on the mythology of goddess Hetheru.

Dua Hetheru Neterit-aah (Adorations to Hathor, the Great Goddess)
Dua Hetheru Sekhem-aah (Adorations to Hathor, the Great Power)
Dua Hetheru Nebt Tawii (Adorations to Hathor, the Mistress of the Earth)
Dua Hetheru Sat Nesu Ra (Adorations to Hathor, the Daughter of King Ra)

A GLOSS ON THE STORY OF HETHERU AND DJEHUTI

The Play, The Enlightenment of Hetheru, is based on the Ancient Egyptian drama known as "The Destruction of Human beings." It is presented in the book "Ushet Rekhat: Worship of the Goddess" by Dr. Muata Ashby. The following is a gloss on the most important aspects of the myth, relating to its spiritual and psycho-mythical implications for the performers.

The Goddess Het-Her (Hetheru)

In a text from the Temple at Dier al-Medina, in Egypt, Hetheru is referred to as having the same divine attributes as Horus. She is described as *"The Golden One"* and *"The Queen of the Gods"*. Her shrines being even more numerous than those of Horus, Hetheru or *Het-Heru*, meaning *"The House of Horus"* and *"The House Above (sky),"* became identified, like Horus, with the salvation of the initiate. In the *Egyptian Book of Coming Forth By Day,* she is the one who urges the initiate to do battle with the monster Apep so as not to lose his / her heart as she cries out: *"Take your armor."* In a separate papyrus, the initiate is told that she (Hetheru) is the one who:

> *"will make your face perfect among the Gods; she will open your eye so that you may see every day... she will make your legs able to walk with ease in the Underworld, Her name is Hetheru, Lady of Amenta."*

Hetheru represents the power of the Ra (Supreme Spirit), therefore, associating with her implies coming into contact with the boundless source of energy which sustains the universe. Making contact with Hetheru implies the development of inner will-power which engenders clarity of vision that will lead to the discernment of what is righteous and what is unrighteous. A mind which is constantly distracted and beset with fetters (anger, hatred, greed, conceit, covetousness, lust, selfishness, etc.) cannot discern the optimal course in life. It becomes weak willed because the negative emotions and feelings drain the mental energy, thus unrighteous actions and sinful thoughts arise and the weak mind cannot resist them. Unrighteous actions lead to adverse situations, and adverse situations lead to pain and sorrow in life. (see *The Asarian Resurrection* and *Egyptian Tantra Yoga* for more on Hetheru and the teachings of Egyptian Tantra Yoga)

In mystical philosophy, the eyes are understood to be the seat of waking consciousness. When you wake someone, you look at their eyes to see if they are awake. The right Eye in particular is seen as the dynamic aspect of consciousness, and Hetheru, as the right Eye of Ra, symbolizes exactly that concept. God (Ra) has projected consciousness (the Eye) into creation, and in so doing, the eye (waking consciousness) becomes involved in various activities within the world of time and space. Similarly, the human soul has projected its image into time and space (the ocean of creation), and in so doing, the psycho-physical self has emerged and human experience is possible. From this process arises the possibility of karmic involvement as well as ignorance and egoism. Karma is the egoistic entanglement in the world and the forgetfulness of one's true nature.

THE MAIN GODS AND GODDESSES OF THE JOURNEY OF HETHERU MYTH

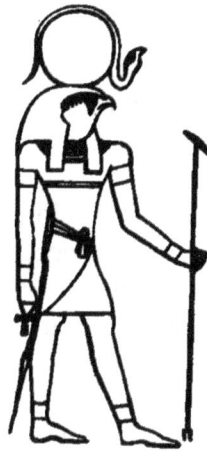 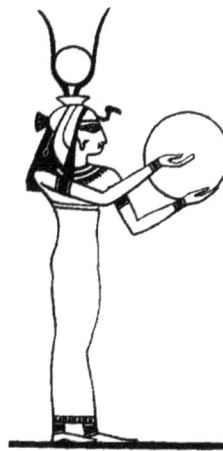

Ra   Hetheru

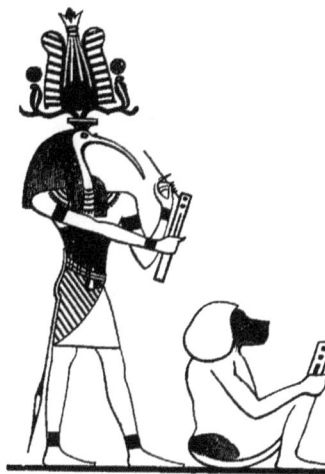   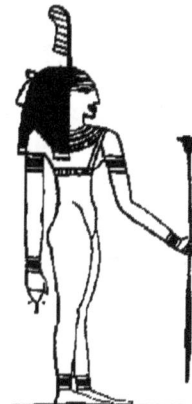

Djehuti as Ibis   Maat

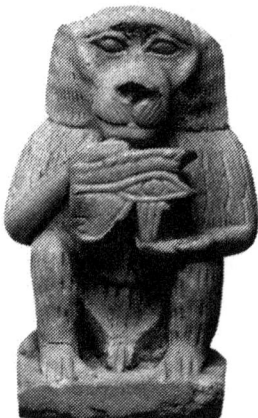

The God Djehuti in the form of a baboon, holding the eye (Hetheru), which he has just cured from its illness (delusion).

Hetheru as a Metaphor

Hetheru represents the predicament of human life. From a state of unity with the Divine (Ra) she becomes degraded to the point of forgetting her true identity. She engages in violent acts and lives out of the lower nature and base desires. This is known as the state of *Dullness of Mind*. The more a person separates from their essential nature, the more a person slides downward into egoism and the lower aspects of the mind which include vices such as anger, hatred, greed, lust, jealousy, etc. Oftentimes these feelings are so strong that they cloud the intellect and render a person incapable of higher forms of thought or feeling. In her aspect as the Eye of Ra Hetheru is the highest power and she is the object of awe and admiration for all. But when her mind was degraded, the same awesome power became the object of tremendous fear because it was uncontrolled and destructive.

Once again, all human beings have the power to act with great goodness or with extreme evil intent. If a person acts out of Maat (virtues such as compassion, non-violence, truth, universal love, harmony, sharing, etc.), then their capacity for goodness is boundless. However, if a person acts out of vices (listed above), then their capacity for negativity is immense even to the extent of self-destruction. When negativity becomes so powerful in the mind, the power of thinking is not the only aspect that becomes impaired. A person's memory and identity becomes impaired as well. Instead of seeing herself as the beautiful goddess of light, and the enforcer of truth and justice, Hetheru saw herself as the vicious wildcat of death. In the same manner people have forgotten their identity as gods and goddesses and have come to regard themselves as miserable human beings caught in the struggle of life for survival and in competition with other human beings and with nature itself.

Djehuti took on the task of saving Hetheru from the pit of negativity and ignorance which she had fallen into. Djehuti represents the intellect, right thinking and truth.

Sebai Djehuti

Djehuti is the god or cosmic principle of learning, writing, mathematics and language. Djehuti is referred to as Thoth by the Greeks. In Ancient Egyptian mythology, he is the scribe of the gods. He appears as the record keeper of the dead in the Books of Coming Forth By Day. He is the patron of learning and of the arts. He is the inventor of writing, and in the specific theology related to him he is also seen as creator of the universe. Djehuti is depicted as a man with the head of a baboon or of an Ibis bird. He also bears pen and ink, and sometimes also the lunar disk and crescent moon.

The ibis is a wading bird related to the stork and the heron. The choice of the ibis indicates a unique feature or quality which spiritual learning requires. This quality is related to the *wading* nature of the Ibis. Wading means *walking in or through a substance, as water, that offers resistance, impedes or makes movement difficult.*

☽

The crescent moon symbol of Djehuti is a figure of the moon in its first quarter. It has concave and convex edges terminating in points. The crescent moon symbol signifies growing or increasing understanding, reason and spiritual wisdom. Therefore, Djehuti is the embodiment of knowledge. This is one of the reasons why he is said to have created writing. He is also the messenger of Ra who brought the special words of power to Aset in the Asarian Resurrection Story in order to resurrect Heru.

Djehuti represents intellect, the mind and its capacity to cut through (wading through) the myriad of thoughts and concepts (water-ocean of consciousness) in order to get to the truth. The universe is understood to be like an ocean of matter through which Ra sails on his boat in order to sustain Creation. Djehuti is Ra's mind, the cosmic mind, with which Ra moves through the ocean of creation. Thus, the universe is known as an ocean of consciousness called Nu or Nun. The spirit (Ra) uses the cosmic mind (Djehuti) to create the objects and varied forms of creation and maintain order in Creation. Therefore, matter (Creation) is in reality consciousness (Primeval Ocean) which has taken on forms (physical objects) in accordance with the will of the Cosmic Mind. The Cosmic Mind also brings forth learning and knowledge to Creation through the arts, sciences and language. Nothing is invented by human beings. Everything that is created by civilization comes from the Cosmic Mind and not from any individual human being. To believe otherwise would be egoistic thought. The more a person is in tune with the Cosmic Mind, the more knowledge he or she can obtain and the more inner peace and fulfillment a person can experience. The farther away a person gets from the Cosmic Mind through negative actions, ignorance and delusion, the less able a person is to discover goodness, inner peace, knowledge, happiness and health in life.

So Djehuti devises a plan to approach Hetheru. Understanding that she is in a state of intense Dullness he knows that he cannot approach her directly by using his ordinary form and by giving her direct teachings as to the nature of the Self (Ra) and her true identity (Hetheru, the Eye of Ra). So he decides to transform himself into the form of a humble, harmless looking baboon instead of presenting himself in the form of a regal ibis headed divinity. It would be very difficult for an ordinary person to behold and accept the real form of the Divine Self (Supreme Being). Therefore, the indirect means of religion, yoga, symbols, myth and parables are adopted until a spiritual aspirant is ready to have a direct experience. At that time the indirect means are placed aside in order to experience the Divine who transcends all forms, concepts, religions and symbols. So Djehuti decided to present to Hetheru some of the most profound teachings related to the nature of the Self in the form of parables in order to gradually gain her confidence and stimulate her latent memories of her own true glory.

In the beginning, the Spiritual Preceptor must help the individual to somehow turn the anguish and pain experienced as a result of interaction with the world into a desire to rise above it. To this end, a series of techniques and disciplines have been developed over thousands of years. Some of these methods are, myths, parables, mental disciplines, meditation and physical culture (Yoga exercises and development of the internal Life Force). The teacher needs to help the seeker to restructure and channel those energies which arise from disappointment and frustration into a healthy dispassion for the illusoriness of the world and its entanglements. The teacher shows the way to develop spiritual aspiration and self-effort directed at sustaining a viable personal spiritual program or *Sheti*.

119

Djehuti is the quintessential image of the Guru in this story. The word "Guru" is an Indian Sanskrit term meaning "Spiritual Preceptor," a teacher of spiritual truths. A Spiritual Preceptor is a Sage who shows others the way to understand the higher reality beyond the ordinary phenomenal universe. He or she shows others how to discover their true identity and realize their oneness with the Divine, in essence, they are spiritual guides.

In Ancient Egyptian Mythology there are two great Spiritual Preceptors. Djehuti is one of them. He is the wonderful teacher of Hetheru. The other one is Aset. In the Shetaut Asar or The Story of Asar, Aset and Heru otherwise known as the Asarian Resurrection, she is the teacher to her son Heru. She trains him in the arts and sciences and the mystical philosophy of Creation and the nature of the Divine Self. She enables Heru to receive the Divine Vision which she obtained from Ra in the Story of Ra and Aset.

The word *Sebai* is the Ancient Egyptian term meaning "Spiritual Preceptor" or "Spiritual Counselor." A Spiritual Preceptor is not only a person who has attained a high level of internal self-discovery and purity but also a person who is well versed in the scriptural writings or the knowledge of parables and myths along with their mystical implications. He or she also knows the practices which lead a person to spiritual evolution (Yoga disciplines).

In order to impart the spiritual teaching, a teacher sometimes needs to disguise him or herself physically in order to approach students. Sometimes the teaching itself needs to be hidden due to the level of evolution of the student. This is why religion was created with three levels of practice, "Myth, Ritual and Mystical Union." A lesser advanced student may require more veiling than a more advanced student. If the teaching is given directly it may be misunderstood or even repudiated altogether due to the state of mind of the individual. Hence, the student must be properly initiated into the teaching and the proper relationship must be established between teacher and student.

The teacher offers humility and honesty with a beguiling wit, cheerfulness and an uplifting outlook. The teacher brings divine food in the form of teachings which uplift the mind by relieving the burden of pain and sorrow which weighs down the soul of a human being due to ignorance and negativity. The divine food is the taste of divine glory. It is a glimpse of the goal which a student must aspire to experience in its fullness but which is experienced in degrees as the teacher gives the spiritual teaching and as it is assimilated by the student.

The student must learn to respect and trust the teacher. Also, the student must allow the teaching to penetrate deeply within the heart. It is only then that the teaching will have a transformative effect. Hetheru allowed Djehuti's words to penetrate her cold, anguished heart and she began to remember her past glory. This is the process of divine memory wherein she began to regain the remembrance of her true identity. The pain of seeing her current level of existence in comparison with her past glory brought her to tears. This is the common realization of a spiritual aspirant when beginning to understand the truth. "What have I done to come down from the heights of divinity to the limited state of human life and mortal existence? How wretched am I? How degraded am I?" These are the kinds of questions asked by a spiritual aspirant who is beginning to understand the meaning of the spiritual teachings. This form of thinking leads to a resolution to regain one's true glory and to rise up from the degradation of ignorance, "May I find a teacher who can guide me on the path to self-discovery and enlightenment at once!" Thus, Hetheru came to respect Djehuti. She accepted his offering, listened to his teachings and later trusted him with her life.

The first parable imparted the understanding of **Maat** or righteous action and the glory of the Divine. Maat is the order, justice and righteousness of the universe. It is the cause and effect law set up by the Divine to maintain harmony in the universe. Any action performed will bring a reaction to the person performing the action. Thus, positive actions set up a positive karmic basis for positive occurrences in a person's life. Negative actions set up a negative karmic basis for negative occurrences to happen in a person's life. It may not be right away but it will occur at some point in time. Therefore, it is important to perform good deeds in order to promote goodness, peace and harmony in your life. "What you do comes back to you!" This is the Ancient Egyptian **Principle of Meskhenet** (popularly known as The Law of Karma in modern culture).

The goddesses *Shai* (fate or destiny), *Rennenet* (fortune) and *Meskhenet* together form the principle of cause and effect which determines a person's future in accordance with their actions, beliefs, feelings and desires, their karmic basis. Therefore, these deities (cosmic forces set up by the Divine) decree whether or not a person will move forward and attain oneness with the Divine or if they will move backwards and experience degraded states of mind. They determine the next birth (family, country, circumstance, etc.) of an individual. The important thing to understand is that they do not determine a person's fate or destiny. They only carry out the sum total of a person's karmic will.

A person's karmic will is their unconscious resolve, based on their accumulated desires, beliefs and feelings which they have lived by, the karmic basis. So if a person desires wealth and carried out various actions in an attempt to gain wealth, they set up a basis for seeking wealth. These actions become stored in the unconscious mind as impressions and at the time of death they impel a person to continue searching for wealth in an unconscious way. If a person was evil in life their own karmic basis will send them to a plane of consciousness where they will experience evil. This is known as Hell. If a person was a performer of good deeds in life their own karmic basis will send them to a plane of consciousness where they will experience heavenly conditions. This is known as Heaven. If the person could not attain some desire in the present lifetime, Meskhenet will cause that person to be reborn in a country, family and circumstance where they will be able to continue pursuing that desire (karmic will). This form of desiring leads to reincarnation and the attainment of things which are ultimately perishable. Heaven and hell are not permanent states of being for the soul. Like the physical world and human life, heaven and hell are relative states. All relative states of experience are transitory. They all come to an end. The only state of being that is permanent and , imperishable is when the mind is enlightened and the eternal Divine Self is discovered. This is because all desires and the entire karmic basis is dissolved. Enlightenment dissolves the karmic basis because it is made up of illusions, desires, passions and ignorance. Since spiritual practice and enlightenment eradicates ignorance and illusions there are no desires left for that which is negative or for the ephemeral pleasures and attainments of mortal existence. If a person was a practitioner of Yoga in life their own purified karmic basis will send them to expand beyond desires and to discover the Divine Self. This is known as spiritual enlightenment, liberation, eternal freedom, immortality, etc.

Therefore, spiritual philosophy directs a spiritual aspirant to desire after that which is not perishable and fleeting, the Divine Self. So it is important to understand that a person can control his or her own fate by controlling their desires, thoughts and feelings. These put together comprise what is referred to as "mind" in mystical philosophy. Therefore, control of the mind is the most important aspect of spiritual practice because the mind determines everything that happens in life, whether it be positive or negative. Mind is the cause of experiences of hell or heaven, happiness or sorrow, enlightenment or degradation, etc.

Even the most infinitesimal forms of life in the universe cannot escape from this karmic law of destiny which is produced by a creature's own actions and desires. Therefore, a spiritual aspirant must learn to desire what is true and to act according to what is good and righteous. The karmic law is an example of the power and glory of the Divine Self (Ra). Even more wonderful is the realization that every living being is a part of the intricate fabric of life and that all are looked after by the Supreme Being, no matter how insignificant they may seem to be. Also, another important teaching here is that no one can get away with evil doing. At some point there is punishment meted for those who transgress the universal laws of life which include compassion, honesty, justice, righteousness, peace and universal love.

Following the first parable, Djehuti introduces the teachings related to the creation of the universe. He explains that from a Primeval Ocean which was formless in the beginning the land of Egypt was created by her father (Ra) and that it is a land of wonders and incomparable beauty. This description is a mystical way of relating the nature of creation and the glory of the entity who created it. Then Djehuti begins to show her that the splendor of the Supreme Being is also her own splendor and glory. He begins to relate her to the Divine Glory that is latent within herself and to bolster her pride in her own heritage. He imparts to her the feeling of goodness that is the Divine. He related how her absence left a great void in Creation and that it caused pain and sorrow to all people. Every life form has a place in Creation. Also, every life form is loved by God who is in the form of relatives, acquaintances and nature itself. So all people have a purpose in life and their existence is meaningful. Also, they are cared for by the Divine Self in various forms. The highest purpose is to discover your true identity and to find your own place which has been decreed for you by the Supreme Divinity.

THE CREATION

The process of creation is explained in the form of a cosmological system for better understanding. Cosmology is a branch of philosophy dealing with the origin, processes, and structure of the universe. Cosmogony is the astrophysical study of the creation and evolution of the universe. Both of these disciplines are inherent facets of Egyptian philosophy through the main religious systems or Companies of the gods and goddesses. A company of gods and goddesses is a group of deities which symbolize a particular cosmic force or principle which emanates from the all-encompassing Supreme Being, from which they have emerged. The Self or Supreme Being manifests creation through the properties and principles represented by the *Pautti* Company of gods and goddesses-cosmic laws of nature. The system or company of gods and goddesses of Anu is regarded as the oldest, and forms the basis of the Osirian Trinity. It is expressed in the diagram below.

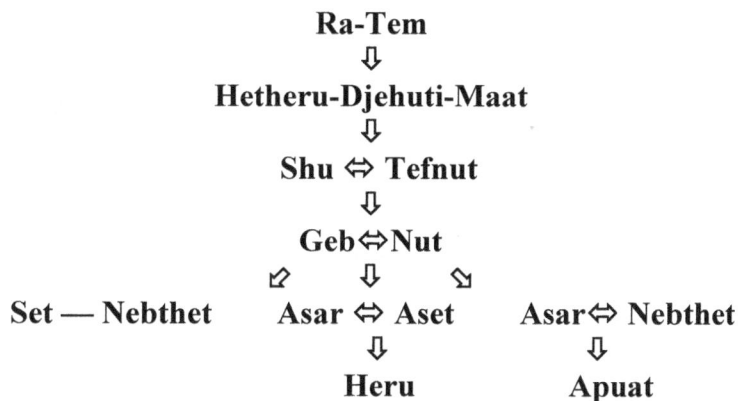

Ra-Tem
⇩
Hetheru-Djehuti-Maat
⇩
Shu ⇔ Tefnut
⇩
Geb⇔Nut
↖   ⇩   ↘
Set — Nebthet   **Asar ⇔ Aset**   **Asar⇔ Nebthet**
⇩   ⇩
Heru   **Apuat**

The diagram above shows that *Psedjet* (Ennead), or the creative principles which are embodied in the primordial gods and goddesses of creation, emanated from the Supreme Being. Ra or Ra-Tem arose out of the *"Nu"*, the Primeval waters, the hidden essence, and began sailing the *"Boat of Millions of Years"* which included the company of gods and goddesses. On his boat emerged the "Neteru" or cosmic principles of creation. The neters of the Ennead are Ra-Atum, Shu, Tefnut, Geb, Nut, Asar, Aset, Set, and Nebthet. Hetheru, Djehuti and Maat represent attributes of the Supreme Being as the very *stuff* or *substratum* which makes up creation. Shu, Tefnut, Geb, Nut, Asar (Osiris), Aset (Isis), Set, and Nebthet (Nephthys) represent the principles upon which creation manifests. Apuat or Anpu (Anubis) is not part of the Ennead. He represents the feature of intellectual discrimination in the Osirian myth. "Sailing" signifies the beginning of motion in creation. Motion implies that events occur in the realm of time and space, thus, the phenomenal universe comes into existence as a mass of moving essence we call the elements. Prior to this motion, there was the primeval state of being without any form and without existence in time or space.

Below: The Tree (Company) of Gods and Goddesses of Anu.

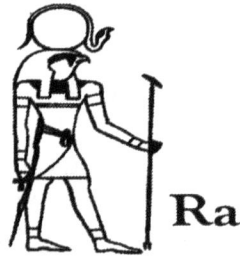

Ra

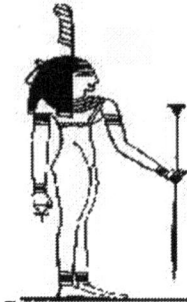 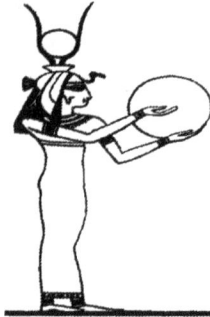 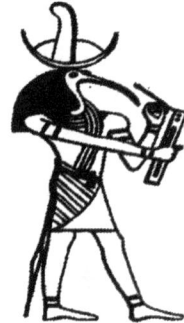

Maat   Hetheru   Djehuti

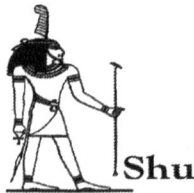 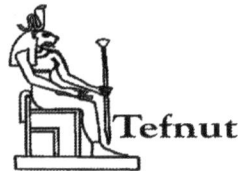

Shu   Tefnut

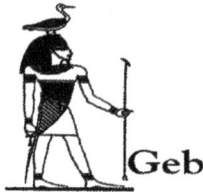 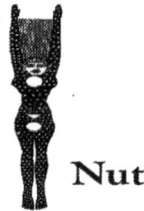

Geb   Nut

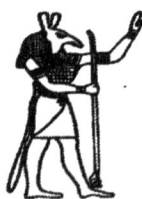 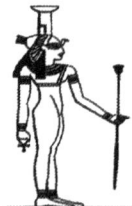   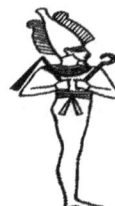 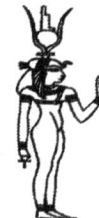

Set   Nebthet   Asar   Aset

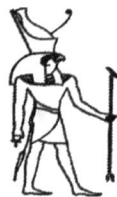

Heru

Hetheru began to cry upon realizing what she seemed to have lost and forgotten about. Then a strange thing happened. Djehuti tried to get her to return to Egypt and all of a sudden she realized what he was doing and she fell back into the pit of negativity. This is not an uncommon occurrence in spiritual life or in ordinary life. Sometimes a person may feel joy and for no reason they may fall into the pits of depression. Sometimes the mental delusion and the erupting emotions cause a person to strike out in anger in an uncontrolled way even towards those who mean goodness to them or those who are speaking truth. This is a factor caused by negative impressions in the karmic basis from the past. Rage is a form of mental illness and its intensity most times incapacitates a person's faculty of self-control. At this time, understanding, gentleness, forgiveness and humility but most of all patience are needed in order to deal with people who are in this degraded, dull state of mind.

Djehuti is the embodiment of patience and the wellspring of parables. So he wisely humbled himself and begged for mercy. He submitted to her power and did not attempt to confront it since he was no match for her might. He cleverly captivated her attention away from anger and violence by channeling her feelings towards interest in another mystical parable. Many times it is necessary to, as it were, trick the mind into listening to the teachings. *Listening to the teachings* is the first and most important step in imparting the spiritual teachings. Therefore, many intriguing, fascinating and beguiling ways have been devised by the Sages to transmit the teachings that captivate the attention of the listener. These are called myths and parables. Myths and parables have a very important feature. They are easier to recall and they have a more direct impact on the untrained mind than direct mystical philosophy because they are easy to identify with as opposed to proverbs or aphorisms which contain raw spiritual truths that require a well trained mind in order to be grasped and appreciated. The next step in the process of learning the teachings it *Reflecting* upon them. This implies the continuous study and practice of the teachings. As you read over a spiritual text and practice its wisdom in your life you will gradually reveal deeper and deeper aspects of the teaching and it will purify your heart in greater and greater degrees. The next step in learning the teachings is *Meditating* upon them. Meditation implies going deep within your mind to a level which is beyond thoughts. It is discovering the *Intuitional* level of mind. The correct understanding of the teachings and their continuous practice in day to day life will automatically lead a person to the meditative state in the course of time. This level of mind is also known in Ancient Egyptian terminology as *Nrutef* or the place where there are no thoughts or vibrations. This practice means communing with the absolute Self within you which is beyond your thoughts, desires and sentimental feelings.

The second parable reinforced the teaching of Ra's omniscience. Hetheru was able to develop *Devotion Towards the Divine.* Devotion towards the Divine is an important development in spiritual life. It means channeling one's emotions towards what is true, beautiful and good and turning away from that which is erroneous, illusory and the source of pain and sorrow in life. So Devotion to God means turning away from the sentimental desires of the ego and turning towards the feelings towards the Divine. *Devotion and Wisdom* are closely related. Each fulfills the other and together they lead a spiritual aspirant to discover the Higher Self. In order to love something you must learn about it. The Divine Self is no exception. The blossoming devotion in Hetheru's heart (Love for God) and the teaching of Djehuti (Wisdom of the Self) allowed Hetheru to calm down and to see the infinite glory of the Divine Self. His teachings revealed the hierarchical order of living beings in Creation and also the idea that even the most powerful living beings are all under the control of and ultimately answer to the Supreme Self.

In the role of Divine avenger or the Divinity who enforces the Divine Law, Djehuti presents the character of the griffin. The griffin is a mythological animal encompassing the body of a lion, the head and wings of an eagle, and the tail of a lion or a serpent. In legends from India, the Far East, and ancient Scythia, griffins were known as the guardians of treasures and mines. In Greek mythology they were the guardians of gold treasures and they drew the carriage or chariot of the sun. In this parable the griffin represents the supreme instrument or power of the Divine. In reality, this is Hetheru's true identity as the Eye of Ra. This is why Djehuti created an elaborate story detailing the hierarchy of creatures and showing how none can escape from the power of the griffin. So in a subtle and indirect way he is teaching her about herself throughout the story and at the end of the parable he reveals to her that she has this same power and that she herself is the Eye of Ra which has power over all creatures. Thus, he introduces her to her own higher nature in a clever and artistic manner.

Another important lesson presented to Hetheru in the first two parables was *faith.* The teaching has showed her how God exists in the very fabric of Creation. In fact all Creation has proceeded from God and every part of Creation is permeated by God's presence. His fairness and compassion is evident in the principles of righteousness, fortune, destiny and cause and effect (Maat, Rennenet, Shai and Meskhenet) which sustain Creation. Also, in order to receive this teaching she needed to develop faith in her teacher. This enabled her to listen and reflect upon the teaching instead of rejecting the teachings and killing the teacher.

The third parable has important implications for spiritual life. Hetheru now has turned away from the pit of negativity, the Dull state of mind, but she is not free from the delusion of ignorance which is rooted deep within her heart. She still remains in the form of a wildcat and even though she has had certain glimpses of the Divine Glory of her Higher Self, she is still partially entangled in the lower self as well. This is the predicament of many people. They have some inkling of their higher spiritual essence but they are caught up in the negativity which still remains to be cleansed from their mind in the form of ignorance, lower desires and wrong thinking. This state is known as *Agitation of Mind*. It is characterized by impure thoughts and feelings based on ignorance of the higher spiritual reality and on indulgence in feelings of egoism, selfishness and individuality. When the mind is agitated, it cannot understand or feel clearly. The thoughts and feelings are tainted with illusion and desire. This is why, when strong emotions and feelings take control of the mind, the mind cannot reason objectively. Likewise, when people are deeply involved in worldly activities with an egoistic intent they are actually moving away from self-discovery and intensifying the illusions, distractions, and worldly desires in their minds. It is like going to the beach and staying at the surface and being aware only of the waves and never going down below the surface to experience the peace and calm below. Conversely, when a person lives in accordance with the teaching and affirms the spiritual reality in all areas of life and when they promote harmony, peace and truth in their life they are moving closer to self-discovery. They may have an active life and still experience inner peace and the divine presence. This is the ideal.

When the mind is calm, it can see the truth clearly and one's idea about oneself also becomes clear as well. A person may feel great in the morning, full of anticipation and cheerfulness because they believe they will make money that day. So his mind is agitated with the expectation of making money and the myriad of things he will do with it. He is not thinking about the possibility of not getting what he wants. This person has deluded himself into expecting a desire to be fulfilled. In the afternoon his expectation was not met so the frustration has set in and depression ensues. He becomes angry and belligerent because he has attached himself to the roller coaster of emotions and egoistic expectation based on the activities he performs in the world of human experience. He is detached from the world of the spirit so he has no awareness of the higher reality. He is like a boat caught up in a storm going up with elation and down with depression with no end in sight. Agitation arises from desires. Desires exist in the mind because it is searching to fulfill a deep longing for wholeness. The mind is erroneously operating based on the concept that acquiring something, entering into a relationship with someone or experiencing some kind of pleasure will fulfill the need, but all activities in the relative world cannot satisfy the need because all activities there are transitory and the mind itself is transitory. It is not possible to experience abiding peace, happiness and joy with something that is transitory, unpredictable and ever-changing.

A spiritual aspirant learns to understand the hollowness of emotions and the futility of worry, pleasure-seeking, wealth, fame and sentimental egoistic values of society and popular culture. A spiritual aspirant is not caught up in them, nor does an aspirant indulge in expectations and desires based on illusion, but those based on reason and truth. Impure thoughts may not necessarily be evil thoughts. They can be based on ignorance alone even if their outcome appears to be evil. The root cause of impurity in the mind is ignorance of the Higher Self. Examples of impure thoughts may be, "I am alone in this world and nobody cares for me," or "I am a miserable human being and there may be a God but he does not care for me," or "Life is for pleasure and I will get mine any way I can and I don't care about anyone else," or "Life has no purpose so don't care whether I live or die."

A spiritual aspirant must learn to think positively and to have positive expectations and desires. These will lead to freedom from negativity and ultimately to the experience of enlightenment. A positive expectation may be to look forward to the experience of discovering God. These are positive expectations in accord with the teachings. An example of a positive desire is to desire to help humanity or save nature or visit a spiritual center, or the desire to read a spiritual text.

The spiritual teaching shows the fallacy of ignorant and egoistic thinking and the manner in which it degrades the mind to the extent of causing people to act callously and selfishly. When a person acts in negative ways, he or she is in reality going against their inner nature, the higher truth deep down. This acts as a poison in one's mind and body which manifests as physical diseases or as mental diseases such as agitation, restlessness, arguing nature, selfishness, etc. When the problem becomes acute, advanced mental and physical diseases arise such as schizophrenia, dementia, delusions, hallucinations and ulcers, cancers, etc. Ultimately, the affliction of negativity in the mind leads to the disease of negative karma, hellish conditions and reincarnation.

So Djehuti tells Hetheru the parable of the two jackals who were spared by the lion because of their *calmness and truthfulness*. Calmness is an important quality for a spiritual aspirant. It implies remaining balanced in the time when there is temptation or when there is disturbance in the environment. It means maintaining an equal vision towards all things and not letting one's emotions hold sway when a decision needs to be made. It means controlling the emotions and desires and not allowing them to control one's life. It means living in accordance with truth and reason and holding fast to correct action even when the mind and body desires something else. In Ancient Egyptian Maat Philosophy (See the book *The Wisdom of Maati* by Dr. Muata Ashby.) this practice is referred to as "keeping the balance." Calmness of mind implies developing equal vision or impartiality. This means not being affected by the ever-changing situations and circumstances of life, be they positive or negative. It means cultivating positive desires and then remaining centered in one's own self, neither expecting fulfillment of desires nor expecting that they will not be fulfilled, but surrendering to the divine will who knows what is best. It is the art of remaining neutral in all conditions and knowing that the Divine will provide the appropriate result for all actions performed. This discipline also involves drawing inner satisfaction from a job well done and allowing the Divine to flow through you for the betterment of all humanity instead of looking to fulfill a personal desire, fruit or reward for what you have done. The discipline of calmness means remaining balanced when things are going well and also when they do not seem to be going well, knowing that God has everything well in hand and that whatever the outcome may be, you will never lose God, eternity and immortality. It is understanding that even if the Divine Self brings you some situation that appears to be negative, that it is ultimately for your greater benefit and spiritual enlightenment. A person who has advanced in calming the mind can experience oneness with God, who is the source of peace and bliss, at any time and in any place.

Truthfulness is important because life is meaningless without it. Without truth nothing real can be known. If a person lives their life in accordance with ignorance and egoism everything they experience will be an illusion. Consequently, they will never be able to discover true happiness and inner peace. For example, most people believe that if they win a lottery they will be happy. This is an ignorant understanding. Their wealth gained from the lottery will only lead to more mental agitation and frustrations later on. However, if they were to understand that true happiness comes from discovering the Higher Self who is infinite peace, immortality and eternity and who has the power to overcome all obstacles, then and only then would they discover true happiness and true wealth.

The fourth parable relates to *humility*. Humility is a quality that should not be confused with humiliation. It is an advanced quality which allows a person to rise above the lower self by sublimating the negative aspects of the ego. Think about it. You may know people or may even remember yourself acting in egoistic ways based on pride in your own physical prowess, strength, beauty, possessions, fame, etc. These egoistic patterns have been developed as you grew up in society and accepted its values which emphasize physical beauty, sexuality, fame, wealth and so on. But if these values are correct, why is it that the people who have the most money, fame, opportunity for sex relations, plastic surgery and notoriety in the world are not the happiest people in the world? Why is it that they are susceptible to the same failings, misfortunes and calamities as all other people? There is a great illusion in popular society that most people follow without examining it closely, that there is some situation or possession or a person in the world that can bring happiness. People have been searching for this since the beginning of time without any success. Hetheru searched for it in vain. She realized that what she was searching for was something she already had within herself. No person or living creature can escape Meskhenet or the jaws of death. This must be clearly understood.

Your ego is not a real part of your personality. It is an illusion which you are sustaining due to an error in understanding your true Higher Self. Your ego, meaning your personality, sense organs, the physical body and your thoughts are in reality transient aspects of your self. They are instruments that the soul assumes in order to have experiences in the world of time and space. They are not absolute realities. This is why at the time of death the soul sheds the personality and the ego, and moves on to other experiences. It may reincarnate at some point in the future and use a new ego personality, just as a person may change clothing. When you act in accordance with righteousness, you are also putting down the ego. When the ego is not given prominence in the personality, it becomes an instrument instead of an obstruction. It becomes a servant instead of a slave master who forces a person to enter into situations and entanglements which at the beginning seem to promise happiness, but which later will lead to great pain and sorrow.

When a person overlooks the correct action in favor of indulging in the personal desires, their actions will be based on egoism. All actions tainted with egoism will inevitably lead to disappointment and frustration at some point in the future. Therefore, the inability to act in accordance with truth must be understood as a defect in the personality, a mental illness. It is the illness of *delusion*. Delusion is intensified by activities which bolster the ego, spiritual ignorance and the egoistic desires. So the pleasure-seeking mentality, the pursuit of sensual pleasures, the desire to possess objects, wealth, fame and power for personal aggrandizement are all examples of egoistic desires which lead to delusion and mental agitation.

The spiritual teaching allows a person to discover a higher forms of fulfillment. It allows a person to understand the underlying basis of Creation and the illusoriness of fleeting egoistic pursuits and desiring perishable objects. You may need to have relationships and possessions in the course of a normal life. However, you should never hold onto anything in the world even as you are experiencing it and possessing it. Your possessions and relationships should be based on righteousness and truth and never on egoism, greed and lust.

The spiritual lifestyle allows a spiritual aspirant to go beyond the erroneous desires, thoughts and feelings that cause agitation of the mind. It shows a person how to calm the mind. When the mind is calmed it becomes clear just as a lake becomes clear when the waves subside. This calmness or serenity of mind allows the real essence of a person to become visible and the ego becomes transparent. When the mind is cleansed the Divine Self comes into clear view as the reality sustaining the ego. When the mind is purified, devoid of the pressure of desires and illusions and a person reaches a state of harmony with the universe, the state of consciousness which a person experiences is referred to as *lucidity of mind*. Lucidity is the quality which is characterized by detachment from the ego and identification with the Higher Self, God. Therefore, lucidity of mind is the objective of all spiritual disciplines because it leads to spiritual enlightenment or self-knowledge and freedom from ignorance, egoism and negative karma. A person who is Lucid is free from attachments and is internally fulfilled. He or she expresses goodwill towards all and display a *gentle nature*. This was Hetheru's condition when she and entered the city of Waset.

It is notable that Hetheru was a vicious beast when she was in the state of Dullness and Agitation, but then she reverted back to her true form when she became gentle, kind and calm. This points to the fact that the source of ugliness and the negativity within the human personality lies in the state of mind which a person adopts. The mindset which a person adopts is in accordance with their level of spiritual evolution. Therefore, spiritual ignorance and delusion lead to ugliness and negativity in the form of anger, hatred, greed, selfishness, jealousy, conflict, frustration and violence.

Detachment from the ego should not be a hard concept to understand. Most people's concept of self is based on their identification with the ego. This is because the ego, its desires, longings and beliefs are all that the person understands. However, spiritual practice allows a person to discover the underlying essence of the mind. This occurs to every person in the world every single day of their lives albeit indirectly. When you go to sleep you experience dreams, but at other times there are no dreams and no awareness of the world. What happened to your ego? It dissolved into your consciousness just as a wave subsides into the ocean from which it arose. When you wake up you are refreshed and you remember a transcendental feeling, but not specifically what happened. What would happen if you were to cause the waves of thoughts and egoistic desires to subside while you were in the state of wakefulness? You would discover in a conscious way, the same truth that you experience in deep dreamless sleep, that there is a deeper part of yourself which sustains your personality and your day to day realities which manifest as the three states of consciousness (Dullness, Agitation and Lucidity) and the seven manifestations of psycho-spiritual consciousness. This is your Higher Self, that part of you which is not dependent on the world and the desires of the ego. When you discover this state of consciousness you are freed from the lower states. You become an enlightened Sage, a knower of the true meaning of the teachings and the monarch or ruler over every aspect of your personality. You become supremely peaceful, *Hetep,* and you rise above all temptations and all illusions. The Higher Self is to be discovered by the following plan as presented in the story of Hetheru and Djehuti. They have been discussed at length throughout this Gloss and are presented summarily below. Even though the principles from the Story of Hetheru and Djehuti have been presented below as a succession in a hierarchical order, all of these disciplines are best practiced in an integral fashion. This means that you do not wait to perfect Maat before starting to practice detachment. You should practice all of these as life presents you with opportunities to test your spiritual strength or Hetheru faculty.

SPIRITUAL ENLIGHTENMENT

↑

Detachment

↑

Humility

↑

Calmness, Truthfulness and Gentleness

↑

Devotion To The Divine

↑

Wisdom: Listening, Reflection and Meditation

↑

Reference and respect for the Spiritual Teacher

↑

Preceptorship - Association with an authentic Spiritual Teacher

↑

Practice Maat and live in accordance with the Principle of Meskhenet

↑

Spiritual Ignorance: Dullness and Agitation

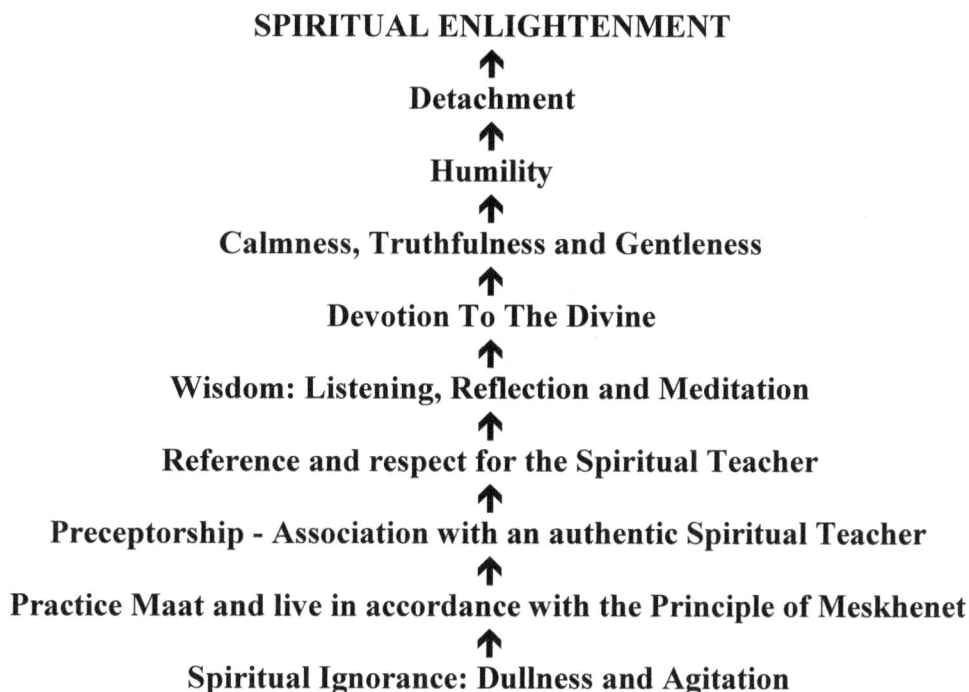

An ordinary person needs to enjoy the company of another person or they need to experience some situation in time and space in order to feel joy and happiness. This is the difference between an un-enlightened person and a person who is advancing spiritually. A person who has experienced the absolute state of consciousness can remember the experience and feel unobstructed bliss and joy. This act of recalling the experience of the Divine is known as remembrance of God. When the feeling of oneness with the Divine becomes the perpetual experience, that person is referred to as one who has attained spiritual enlightenment or oneness with the Divine. Ordinary people experience glimpses of this bliss and joy. However, they ascribe it to some object they acquired or to some person in their life or to some situation they saw as beneficial. Others experience joy spontaneously for no apparent reason, but it fades away as mysteriously as it came. A Sage (practitioner of Yoga) learns to discover the source of bliss or unobstructed joy and abides there continuously by not allowing egoistic desires, expectations, sentimentality, anger, hatred, greed, etc., to cloud their experience. The unobstructed experience of joy and peace is what all living things are striving for in various ways, even if they do not realize it. Therefore, it is said that an enlightened Sage has accomplished the most important task in life, achieving which, nothing is left to be achieved.

The character of Djehuti and his relationship to Hetheru implies another important teaching in relation to the teacher-student relationship. An advanced spiritual teacher does not see him or herself as the originator of the teaching. It is God who is working through them to bring the teaching forth for the benefit of all humanity. People often ask where God is when bad things are happening and why there is no one to help in time of need. People need to understand that God is everywhere, especially in the heart of authentic spiritual preceptors and in the good intentions of others. However, people need to purify their hearts because with an impure heart that is constantly producing negative thoughts and feelings they will constantly lead themselves into negative situations and relationships. Also, if they are impure they would not benefit from the teachings even if the greatest spiritual teachers such as Djehuti, Aset, Jesus, Buddha, etc. were present. Therefore, the compassion of God is so great that she has come to the world in the form of the scriptural writings, compassion and the spirit of service in the human heart, the Sages and Saints, and the high mystical philosophy and religious iconography.

There is also a mystical significance to the rejoicing in the cities when Hetheru returned to her rightful place. The cities mentioned, Anu, Het-ku-Ptah and Waset, relate to cities of the gods of the Great Ancient Egyptian Trinity of *Amun-Ra-Ptah*. The Ancient Egyptian Hymns of Amun contain the key to understanding the mystical meaning of the teaching. The Ancient Egyptian teaching "Neberdjer-Amun-Ra-Ptah" is explained as follows. Neberdjer means the "Supreme Being." Amun-Ra-Ptah represent the triune manner in which the Supreme Being manifests creation. Amun represents witnessing consciousness or self-awareness. Ra represents the cosmic mind which sustains all mental activity and the means for consciousness to interact with Creation, the light or power of consciousness. Ptah represents the physical universe with which the witnessing consciousness interacts. This triad is also related to human life. All human beings have three bodies, "physical, astral and causal." The soul in every human being is like a spark of the Self, Neberdjer, who uses these bodies in order to have experiences in the varied forms of life in Creation.

The Trinity also relates to the human mind. The mind of a human being experiences three states of awareness, "waking, dream and dreamless sleep" as well as three modes of manifestation, "dullness, agitation and lucidity." Thus, the return of Hetheru signifies the rejoicing in all aspects of a person's personality, the emotions, intellect, will and the physical nature. This is, of course, a description of a human being who has attained spiritual perfection.

The seven day festivity relates to the seven centers of psycho-spiritual consciousness. Hetheru is the goddess of the seven aspects of consciousness in her form as the seven Divine Hetheru Cows. The one Supreme Being in the form of a Bull (Asar-Osiris) expresses in seven modes of consciousness (the seven cows). This expression of the spirit is symbolized by Hetheru in her seven aspects. Hetheru represents divine consciousness emanating from the Divine Self (Eye of Ra emanating from the Sun). She (divine consciousness) expresses herself (itself) as the essence which sustains the mind of every human being as well. Every human being has seven psycho-spiritual consciousness centers in their astral body. These act as transducers of psychic energy from the soul level of consciousness and they sustain the physical body. Each center relates to an aspect of human personality and as a person develops **Arat** or the Serpent Power energy (Inner Life Force known as Kundalini in India or Chi in China) of the goddess, these energy centers are cleansed and their power is allowed to unfold. Thus, a human being evolves spiritually through the power of the goddess. The Serpent Power automatically awakens when a person studies and practices the teachings. However, the process of raising one's spiritual power may be aided by specific exercises such as concentration, proper breathing, righteous action, devotion to the Divine, meditation on the meanings of the spiritual symbols and surrendering to the will of the Higher Self (God). These techniques allow a person to transform their waking personality so that they may discover their innermost Self: God. For more on the Serpent Power and the techniques for cultivating it see the book "The Serpent Power" by Dr. Muata Ashby.

May the blessings of Hetheru be with you!

NEW BOOK: **The Glorious Light Meditation Technique of Ancient Egypt**
ISBN: 1-884564-15-1 $12.95 (PB)

New for the year 2000. This volume is based on the earliest known instruction in history given for the practice of formal meditation. Discovered by Dr. Muata Ashby, it is inscribed on the walls of the Tomb of Seti I in Thebes Egypt. This volume details the philosophy and practice of this unique system of meditation originated in Ancient Egypt and the earliest practice of meditation known in the world which occurred in the most advanced African Culture. It is based on the scripture related to the myth of Hetheru and Djehuti, a mythic play from Ancient Egypt.

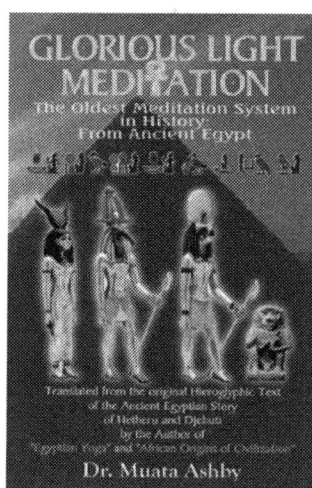

An Ancient Egyptian Play: The Enlightenment of Hetheru Audio Lecture Series
- Now Available: Audio Lectures

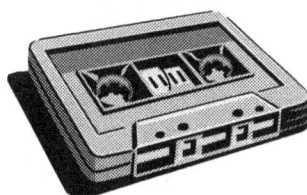

AUDIO
CASSETTE

303 CLASS 2 The Story of Hethor and Djehuti: The Three States of Consciousness - by Author Dr. Muata Ashby $9.99 - 90 min.
4032 Discussion of the teachings contained in the play "The Enlightenment of Hetheru" with readings from the play – Part 1 by Dr. Karen Ashby $9.99
4033 Discussion of the teachings contained in the play "The Enlightenment of Hetheru" with readings from the play – Part 2 by Dr. Karen Ashby $9.99

3012 Dramatic Arts, Music and Enlightenment in Ancient Egyptian Theater and the The Enlightenment of Hetheru: Part 1 $9.99

3012 Dramatic Arts, Music and Enlightenment in Ancient Egyptian Theater and the The Enlightenment of Hetheru: Part 2 $9.99

Sema Institute of Yoga P.O. Box 570459, Miami Fl. 33257

(305)-378-6253.68

Video Presentation Myth of Goddess Hetheru and God Djehuti

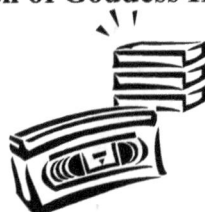

Mysticism of the Myth of Goddess Hetheru and God Djehuti (12/2000) $19.99

Recordings of the music and chants to be used for the Hetheru Play

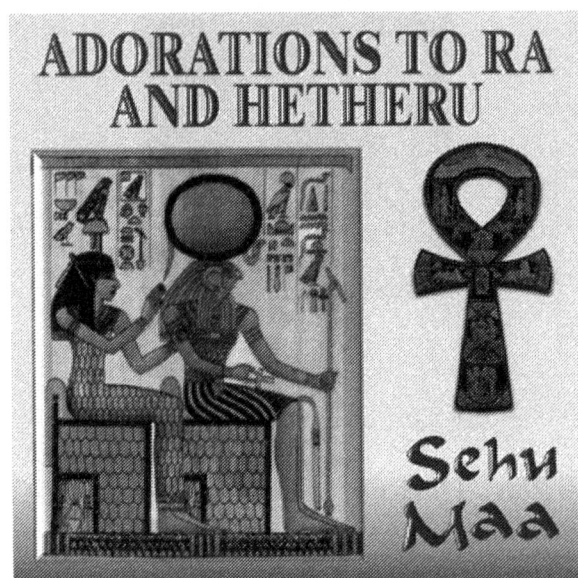

ANORATIONS TO RA AND HETHERU
NEW Egyptian Yoga Music CD
By Seba Maa (Muata Ashby)
Based on the Words of Power of Ra and Hetheru
played on reproductions of Ancient Egyptian Instruments **Ancient Egyptian Instruments used: Voice, Clapping, Nefer Lute, Tar Drum, Sistrums, Cymbals** – The Chants, Devotions, Rhythms and Festive Songs Of the Neteru – Ideal for meditation, and devotional singing and dancing.

©1999 By Muata Ashby
CD $14.99 –Cassette $10
UPC# 761527100221

Other Books From C M Books

P.O.Box 570459
Miami, Florida, 33257
(305) 378-6253 Fax: (305) 378-6253

This book is part of a series on the study and practice of Ancient Egyptian Yoga and Mystical Spirituality based on the writings of Dr. Muata Abhaya Ashby. They are also part of the Egyptian Yoga Course provided by the Sema Institute of Yoga. Below you will find a listing of the other books in this series. For more information send for the Egyptian Yoga Book-Audio-Video Catalog or the Egyptian Yoga Course Catalog.

Now you can study the teachings of Egyptian and Indian Yoga wisdom and Spirituality with the Egyptian Yoga Mystical Spirituality Series. The Egyptian Yoga Series takes you through the Initiation process and lead you to understand the mysteries of the soul and the Divine and to attain the highest goal of life: ENLIGHTENMENT. The *Egyptian Yoga Series*, takes you on an in depth study of Ancient Egyptian mythology and their inner mystical meaning. Each Book is prepared for the serious student of the mystical sciences and provides a study of the teachings along with exercises, assignments and projects to make the teachings understood and effective in real life. The Series is part of the Egyptian Yoga course but may be purchased even if you are not taking the course. The series is ideal for study groups.

Prices subject to change.

1.   EGYPTIAN YOGA: THE PHILOSOPHY OF ENLIGHTENMENT An original, fully illustrated work, including hieroglyphs, detailing the meaning of the Egyptian mysteries, tantric yoga, psycho-spiritual and physical exercises. Egyptian Yoga is a guide to the practice of the highest spiritual philosophy which leads to absolute freedom from human misery and to immortality. It is well known by scholars that Egyptian philosophy is the basis of Western and Middle Eastern religious philosophies such as *Christianity, Islam, Judaism,* the *Kabala,* and Greek philosophy, but what about Indian philosophy, Yoga and Taoism? What were the original teachings? How can they be practiced today? What is the source of pain and suffering in the world and what is the solution? Discover the deepest mysteries of the mind and universe within and outside of your self. 8.5" X 11" ISBN: 1-884564-01-1 Soft $19.95

2.   EGYPTIAN YOGA II: The Supreme Wisdom of Enlightenment by Dr. Muata Ashby ISBN 1-884564-39-9 $23.95 U.S. In this long awaited sequel to *Egyptian Yoga: The Philosophy of Enlightenment* you will take a fascinating and enlightening journey back in time and discover the teachings which constituted the epitome of Ancient Egyptian spiritual wisdom. What are the disciplines which lead to the fulfillment of all desires? Delve into the three states of consciousness (waking, dream and deep sleep) and the fourth state which transcends them all, Neberdjer, "The Absolute." These teachings of the city of Waset (Thebes) were the crowning achievement of the Sages of Ancient Egypt. They establish the standard mystical keys for understanding the profound mystical symbolism of the Triad of human consciousness.

3.   THE KEMETIC DIET: GUIDE TO HEALTH, DIET AND FASTING Health issues have always been important to human beings since the beginning of time. The earliest records of history show that the art of healing was held in high esteem since the time of Ancient Egypt. In the early 20th century, medical doctors had almost attained the status of sainthood by the promotion of the idea that they alone were "scientists" while other healing modalities and traditional healers who did not follow the "scientific method' were nothing but superstitious, ignorant charlatans who at best would take the money of their clients and at worst kill them with the unscientific "snake oils" and "irrational theories". In the late 20th century, the failure of the modern medical establishment's ability to lead the general public to good health, promoted the move by many in society towards "alternative medicine". Alternative medicine disciplines are those healing modalities which do not adhere to the philosophy of allopathic medicine. Allopathic medicine is what medical doctors practice by an large. It is the theory that disease is caused by agencies outside the body such as bacteria, viruses or physical means which affect the body. These can therefore be treated by medicines and therapies The natural healing method began in the absence of extensive technologies with the idea that all the answers for health may be found in nature or rather, the deviation from nature. Therefore, the health of the body can be restored by correcting the aberration and thereby restoring balance. This is the area that will be covered in this volume. Allopathic techniques have their place in the art of healing. However, we should not forget that the body is a grand achievement of the spirit and built into it is the capacity to maintain itself and heal itself. Ashby, Muata ISBN: 1-884564-49-6 $28.95

4.   INITIATION INTO EGYPTIAN YOGA Shedy: Spiritual discipline or program, to go deeply into the mysteries, to study the mystery teachings and literature profoundly, to penetrate the mysteries. You will learn about the mysteries of initiation into the teachings and practice of Yoga and how to become an Initiate of the mystical sciences. This insightful manual is the first in a series which introduces you to the goals of daily spiritual and yoga practices: Meditation, Diet, Words of Power and the ancient wisdom teachings. 8.5" X 11" ISBN 1-884564-02-X   Soft Cover $24.95 U.S.

5.   *THE AFRICAN ORIGINS OF CIVILIZATION, MYSTICAL RELIGION AND YOGA PHILOSOPHY* HARD COVER EDITION ISBN: 1-884564-50-X $80.00 U.S.   81/2" X 11"   Part 1, Part 2, Part 3 in one volume 683 Pages Hard Cover First Edition Three volumes in one. Over the past several years I have been asked to put together in one volume the most important evidences showing the correlations and common teachings between Kamitan (Ancient Egyptian) culture and religion and that of India. The questions of the history of Ancient Egypt, and the latest archeological evidences showing civilization and culture in Ancient Egypt and its spread to other countries, has intrigued many scholars as well as mystics over the years. Also, the possibility that Ancient Egyptian Priests and Priestesses migrated to Greece, India and other countries to carry on the traditions of the Ancient Egyptian Mysteries, has been speculated over the years as well. In chapter 1 of the book *Egyptian Yoga The Philosophy of Enlightenment,* 1995, I first introduced the deepest comparison between Ancient Egypt and India that had been brought forth up to that time. Now, in the year 2001 this new book, *THE AFRICAN ORIGINS OF CIVILIZATION, MYSTICAL RELIGION AND YOGA PHILOSOPHY,* more fully explores the motifs, symbols and philosophical

correlations between Ancient Egyptian and Indian mysticism and clearly shows not only that Ancient Egypt and India were connected culturally but also spiritually. How does this knowledge help the spiritual aspirant? This discovery has great importance for the Yogis and mystics who follow the philosophy of Ancient Egypt and the mysticism of India. It means that India has a longer history and heritage than was previously understood. It shows that the mysteries of Ancient Egypt were essentially a yoga tradition which did not die but rather developed into the modern day systems of Yoga technology of India. It further shows that African culture developed Yoga Mysticism earlier than any other civilization in history. All of this expands our understanding of the unity of culture and the deep legacy of Yoga, which stretches into the distant past, beyond the Indus Valley civilization, the earliest known high culture in India as well as the Vedic tradition of Aryan culture. Therefore, Yoga culture and mysticism is the oldest known tradition of spiritual development and Indian mysticism is an extension of the Ancient Egyptian mysticism. By understanding the legacy which Ancient Egypt gave to India the mysticism of India is better understood and by comprehending the heritage of Indian Yoga, which is rooted in Ancient Egypt the Mysticism of Ancient Egypt is also better understood. This expanded understanding allows us to prove the underlying kinship of humanity, through the common symbols, motifs and philosophies which are not disparate and confusing teachings but in reality expressions of the same study of truth through metaphysics and mystical realization of Self. (HARD COVER)

6. AFRICAN ORIGINS BOOK 1 PART 1 African Origins of African Civilization, Religion, Yoga Mysticism and Ethics Philosophy-Soft Cover $24.95 ISBN: 1-884564-55-0

7. AFRICAN ORIGINS BOOK 2 PART 2 African Origins of Western Civilization, Religion and Philosophy(Soft) -Soft Cover $24.95 ISBN: 1-884564-56-9

8. EGYPT AND INDIA (AFRICAN ORIGINS BOOK 3 PART 3) African Origins of Eastern Civilization, Religion, Yoga Mysticism and Philosophy-Soft Cover $29.95 (Soft) ISBN: 1-884564-57-7

9. THE MYSTERIES OF ISIS: **The Ancient Egyptian Philosophy of Self-Realization** - There are several paths to discover the Divine and the mysteries of the higher Self. This volume details the mystery teachings of the goddess Aset (Isis) from Ancient Egypt- the path of wisdom. It includes the teachings of her temple and the disciplines that are enjoined for the initiates of the temple of Aset as they were given in ancient times. Also, this book includes the teachings of the main myths of Aset that lead a human being to spiritual enlightenment and immortality. Through the study of ancient myth and the illumination of initiatic understanding the idea of God is expanded from the mythological comprehension to the metaphysical. Then this metaphysical understanding is related to you, the student, so as to begin understanding your true divine nature. ISBN 1-884564-24-0 $22.99

10. EGYPTIAN PROVERBS: TEMT TCHAAS *Temt Tchaas* means: collection of ——— Ancient Egyptian Proverbs How to live according to MAAT Philosophy. Beginning

Meditation. All proverbs are indexed for easy searches. For the first time in one volume, ——Ancient Egyptian Proverbs, wisdom teachings and meditations, fully illustrated with hieroglyphic text and symbols. EGYPTIAN PROVERBS is a unique collection of knowledge and wisdom which you can put into practice today and transform your life. 5.5"x 8.5" $14.95 U.S   ISBN: 1-884564-00-3

11.   THE PATH OF DIVINE LOVE The Process of Mystical Transformation and The Path of Divine Love   This Volume focuses on the ancient wisdom teachings of "Neter Merri" –the Ancient Egyptian philosophy of Divine Love and how to use them in a scientific process for self-transformation. Love is one of the most powerful human emotions. It is also the source of Divine feeling that unifies God and the individual human being. When love is fragmented and diminished by egoism the Divine connection is lost. The Ancient tradition of Neter Merri leads human beings back to their Divine connection, allowing them to discover their innate glorious self that is actually Divine and immortal. This volume will detail the process of transformation from ordinary consciousness to cosmic consciousness through the integrated practice of the teachings and the path of Devotional Love toward the Divine. 5.5"x 8.5" ISBN 1-884564-11-9 $22.99

12.   INTRODUCTION TO MAAT PHILOSOPHY: Spiritual Enlightenment Through the Path of Virtue   Known as Karma Yoga in India, the teachings of MAAT for living virtuously and with orderly wisdom are explained and the student is to begin practicing the precepts of Maat in daily life so as to promote the process of purification of the heart in preparation for the judgment of the soul. This judgment will be understood not as an event that will occur at the time of death but as an event that occurs continuously, at every moment in the life of the individual. The student will learn how to become allied with the forces of the Higher Self and to thereby begin cleansing the mind (heart) of impurities so as to attain a higher vision of reality. ISBN 1-884564-20-8 $22.99

13.   MEDITATION The Ancient Egyptian Path to Enlightenment   Many people do not know about the rich history of meditation practice in Ancient Egypt. This volume outlines the theory of meditation and presents the Ancient Egyptian Hieroglyphic text which give instruction as to the nature of the mind and its three modes of expression. It also presents the texts which give instruction on the practice of meditation for spiritual Enlightenment and unity with the Divine. This volume allows the reader to begin practicing meditation by explaining, in easy to understand terms, the simplest form of meditation and working up to the most advanced form which was practiced in ancient times and which is still practiced by yogis around the world in modern times. ISBN 1-884564-27-7 $24.99

14.   THE GLORIOUS LIGHT MEDITATION Technique of Ancient Egypt ISBN: 1-884564-15-1$14.95 (PB) New for the year 2000. This volume is based on the earliest known instruction in history given for the practice of formal meditation. Discovered by Dr. Muata Ashby, it is inscribed on the walls of the Tomb of Seti I in Thebes Egypt. This volume details the philosophy and practice of this unique system of meditation originated

in Ancient Egypt and the earliest practice of meditation known in the world which occurred in the most advanced African Culture.

15. THE SERPENT POWER: The Ancient Egyptian Mystical Wisdom of the Inner Life Force.   This Volume specifically deals with the latent life Force energy of the universe and in the human body, its control and sublimation. How to develop the Life Force energy of the subtle body. This Volume will introduce the esoteric wisdom of the science of how virtuous living acts in a subtle and mysterious way to cleanse the latent psychic energy conduits and vortices of the spiritual body. ISBN 1-884564-19-4 $22.95

16. EGYPTIAN YOGA *The Postures of The Gods and Goddesses* Discover the physical postures and exercises practiced thousands of years ago in Ancient Egypt which are today known as Yoga exercises. This work is based on the pictures and teachings from the Creation story of Ra, The Asarian Resurrection Myth and the carvings and reliefs from various Temples in Ancient Egypt 8.5" X 11" ISBN 1-884564-10-0 Soft Cover $21.95 Exercise video $20

17. EGYPTIAN TANTRA YOGA: The Art of Sex Sublimation and Universal Consciousness This Volume will expand on the male and female principles within the human body and in the universe and further detail the sublimation of sexual energy into spiritual energy. The student will study the deities Min and Hathor, Asar and Aset, Geb and Nut and discover the mystical implications for a practical spiritual discipline. This Volume will also focus on the Tantric aspects of Ancient Egyptian and Indian mysticism, the purpose of sex and the mystical teachings of sexual sublimation which lead to self-knowledge and Enlightenment. 5.5"x 8.5" ISBN 1-884564-03-8 $24.95

18. ASARIAN RELIGION: RESURRECTING OSIRIS The path of Mystical Awakening and the Keys to Immortality NEW REVISED AND EXPANDED EDITION!   The Ancient Sages created stories based on human and superhuman beings whose struggles, aspirations, needs and desires ultimately lead them to discover their true Self. The myth of Aset, Asar and Heru is no exception in this area. While there is no one source where the entire story may be found, pieces of it are inscribed in various ancient Temples walls, tombs, steles and papyri. For the first time available, the complete myth of Asar, Aset and Heru has been compiled from original Ancient Egyptian, Greek and Coptic Texts. This epic myth has been richly illustrated with reliefs from the Temple of Heru at Edfu, the Temple of Aset at Philae, the Temple of Asar at Abydos, the Temple of Hathor at Denderah and various papyri, inscriptions and reliefs. Discover the myth which inspired the teachings of the *Shetaut Neter* (Egyptian Mystery System - Egyptian Yoga) and the Egyptian Book of Coming Forth By Day. Also, discover the three levels of Ancient Egyptian Religion, how to understand the mysteries of the Duat or Astral World and how to discover the abode of the Supreme in the Amenta, *The Other World*   The ancient religion of Asar, Aset and Heru, if properly understood, contains all of the elements necessary to lead the sincere aspirant to attain immortality through inner self-discovery. This volume presents the entire myth and explores the main mystical themes and rituals associated with the myth for understating human existence, creation and the way to achieve spiritual emancipation - *Resurrection.* The Asarian myth is so powerful that it

influenced and is still having an effect on the major world religions. Discover the origins and mystical meaning of the Christian Trinity, the Eucharist ritual and the ancient origin of the birthday of Jesus Christ. Soft Cover ISBN: 1-884564-27-5 $24.95

19. THE EGYPTIAN BOOK OF THE DEAD MYSTICISM OF THE PERT EM HERU $28.95   ISBN# 1-884564-28-3 Size: 8½" X 11" I Know myself, I know myself, I am One With God!–From the Pert Em Heru "The Ru Pert em Heru" or "Ancient Egyptian Book of The Dead," or "Book of Coming Forth By Day" as it is more popularly known, has fascinated the world since the successful translation of Ancient Egyptian hieroglyphic scripture over 150 years ago. The astonishing writings in it reveal that the Ancient Egyptians believed in life after death and in an ultimate destiny to discover the Divine. The elegance and aesthetic beauty of the hieroglyphic text itself has inspired many see it as an art form in and of itself. But is there more to it than that? Did the Ancient Egyptian wisdom contain more than just aphorisms and hopes of eternal life beyond death? In this volume Dr. Muata Ashby, the author of over 25 books on Ancient Egyptian Yoga Philosophy has produced a new translation of the original texts which uncovers a mystical teaching underlying the sayings and rituals instituted by the Ancient Egyptian Sages and Saints. "Once the philosophy of Ancient Egypt is understood as a mystical tradition instead of as a religion or primitive mythology, it reveals its secrets which if practiced today will lead anyone to discover the glory of spiritual self-discovery. The Pert em Heru is in every way comparable to the Indian Upanishads or the Tibetan Book of the Dead." Muata Abhaya Ashby

20. ANUNIAN THEOLOGY THE MYSTERIES OF RA The Philosophy of Anu and The Mystical Teachings of The Ancient Egyptian Creation Myth Discover the mystical teachings contained in the Creation Myth and the gods and goddesses who brought creation and human beings into existence. The Creation Myth holds the key to understanding the universe and for attaining spiritual Enlightenment. ISBN: 1-884564-38-0 40 pages $14.95

21. MYSTERIES OF MIND Mystical Psychology & Mental Health for Enlightenment and Immortality based on the Ancient Egyptian Philosophy of Menefer -Mysticism of Ptah, Egyptian Physics and Yoga Metaphysics and the Hidden properties of Matter.   This volume uncovers the mystical psychology of the Ancient Egyptian wisdom teachings centering on the philosophy of the Ancient Egyptian city of Menefer (Memphite Theology). How to understand the mind and how to control the senses and lead the mind to health, clarity and mystical self-discovery. This Volume will also go deeper into the philosophy of God as creation and will explore the concepts of modern science and how they correlate with ancient teachings. This Volume will lay the ground work for the understanding of the philosophy of universal consciousness and the initiatic/yogic insight into who or what is God? ISBN 1-884564-07-0 $22.95

22. THE GODDESS AND THE EGYPTIAN MYSTERIESTHE PATH OF THE GODDESS THE GODDESS PATH The Secret Forms of the Goddess and the Rituals of Resurrection The Supreme Being may be worshipped as father or as mother. *Ushet Rekhat* or *Mother Worship*, is the spiritual process of worshipping the Divine in the form of the Divine

Goddess. It celebrates the most important forms of the Goddess including *Nathor, Maat, Aset, Arat, Amentet and Hathor* and explores their mystical meaning as well as the rising of *Sirius,* the star of Aset (Aset) and the new birth of Hor (Heru). The end of the year is a time of reckoning, reflection and engendering a new or renewed positive movement toward attaining spiritual Enlightenment. The Mother Worship devotional meditation ritual, performed on five days during the month of December and on New Year's Eve, is based on the Ushet Rekhit. During the ceremony, the cosmic forces, symbolized by Sirius - and the constellation of Orion ---, are harnessed through the understanding and devotional attitude of the participant. This propitiation draws the light of wisdom and health to all those who share in the ritual, leading to prosperity and wisdom. $14.95 ISBN 1-884564-18-6

23. *THE MYSTICAL JOURNEY FROM JESUS TO CHRIST* $24.95   ISBN# 1-884564-05-4 size: 8½" X 11" Discover the ancient Egyptian origins of Christianity before the Catholic Church and learn the mystical teachings given by Jesus to assist all humanity in becoming Christlike. Discover the secret meaning of the Gospels that were discovered in Egypt. Also discover how and why so many Christian churches came into being. Discover that the Bible still holds the keys to mystical realization even though its original writings were changed by the church. Discover how to practice the original teachings of Christianity which leads to the Kingdom of Heaven.

24. THE STORY OF ASAR, ASET AND HERU: An Ancient Egyptian Legend (For Children)   Now for the first time, the most ancient myth of Ancient Egypt comes alive for children. Inspired by the books *The Asarian Resurrection: The Ancient Egyptian Bible* and *The Mystical Teachings of The Asarian Resurrection, The Story of Asar, Aset and Heru* is an easy to understand and thrilling tale which inspired the children of Ancient Egypt to aspire to greatness and righteousness. If you and your child have enjoyed stories like *The Lion King* and *Star Wars you will love The Story of Asar, Aset and Heru.* Also, if you know the story of Jesus and Krishna you will discover than Ancient Egypt had a similar myth and that this myth carries important spiritual teachings for living a fruitful and fulfilling life. This book may be used along with *The Parents Guide To The Asarian Resurrection Myth: How to Teach Yourself and Your Child the Principles of Universal Mystical Religion.* The guide provides some background to the Asarian Resurrection myth and it also gives insight into the mystical teachings contained in it which you may introduce to your child. It is designed for parents who wish to grow spiritually with their children and it serves as an introduction for those who would like to study the Asarian Resurrection Myth in depth and to practice its teachings. 41 pages 8.5" X 11"   ISBN: 1-884564-31-3 $12.95

25. THE PARENTS GUIDE TO THE AUSARIAN RESURRECTION MYTH: How to Teach Yourself and Your Child the Principles of Universal Mystical Religion.   This insightful manual brings for the timeless wisdom of the ancient through the Ancient Egyptian myth of Asar, Aset and Heru and the mystical teachings contained in it for parents who want to guide their children to understand and practice the teachings of mystical spirituality. This manual may be used with the children's storybook *The Story of Asar, Aset and Heru* by Dr. Muata Abhaya Ashby. 5.5"x 8.5"   ISBN: 1-884564-30-5 $14.95

26. HEALING THE CRIMINAL HEART BOOK 1 Introduction to Maat Philosophy, Yoga and Spiritual Redemption Through the Path of Virtue   Who is a criminal? Is there such a thing as a criminal heart? What is the source of evil and sinfulness and is there any way to rise above it? Is there redemption for those who have committed sins, even the worst crimes?   Ancient Egyptian mystical psychology holds important answers to these questions. Over ten thousand years ago mystical psychologists, the Sages of Ancient Egypt, studied and charted the human mind and spirit and laid out a path which will lead to spiritual redemption, prosperity and Enlightenment.   This introductory volume brings forth the teachings of the Asarian Resurrection, the most important myth of Ancient Egypt, with relation to the faults of human existence: anger, hatred, greed, lust, animosity, discontent, ignorance, egoism jealousy, bitterness, and a myriad of psycho-spiritual ailments which keep a human being in a state of negativity and adversity. 5.5"x 8.5"   ISBN: 1-884564-17-8 $15.95

27. THEATER & DRAMA OF THE ANCIENT EGYPTIAN MYSTERIES: Featuring the Ancient Egyptian stage play-"The Enlightenment of Hathor' Based on an Ancient Egyptian Drama, The original Theater -Mysticism of the Temple of Hetheru $14.95   By Dr. Muata Ashby

28. GUIDE TO PRINT ON DEMAND: SELF-PUBLISH FOR PROFIT, SPIRITUAL FULFILLMENT AND SERVICE TO HUMANITY Everyone asks us how we produced so many books in such a short time. Here are the secrets to writing and producing books that uplift humanity and how to get them printed for a fraction of the regular cost. Anyone can become an author even if they have limited funds. All that is necessary is the willingness to learn how the printing and book business work and the desire to follow the special instructions given here for preparing your manuscript format. Then you take your work directly to the non-traditional companies who can produce your books for less than the traditional book printer can. ISBN: 1-884564-40-2 $16.95 U. S.

29. Egyptian Mysteries: Vol. 1, Shetaut Neter ISBN: 1-884564-41-0 $19.99 What are the Mysteries? For thousands of years the spiritual tradition of Ancient Egypt, *Shetaut Neter,* "The Egyptian Mysteries," "The Secret Teachings," have fascinated, tantalized and amazed the world. At one time exalted and recognized as the highest culture of the world, by Africans, Europeans, Asiatics, Hindus, Buddhists and other cultures of the ancient world, in time it was shunned by the emerging orthodox world religions. Its temples desecrated, its philosophy maligned, its tradition spurned, its philosophy dormant in the mystical *Medu Neter,* the mysterious hieroglyphic texts which hold the secret symbolic meaning that has scarcely been discerned up to now. What are the secrets of *Nehast* {spiritual awakening and emancipation, resurrection}. More than just a literal translation, this volume is for awakening to the secret code *Shetitu* of the teaching which was not deciphered by Egyptologists, nor could be understood by ordinary spiritualists. This book is a reinstatement of the original science made available for our times, to the reincarnated followers of Ancient Egyptian culture and the prospect of spiritual freedom to break the bonds of *Khemn,* "ignorance," and slavery to evil forces: *Såaa .*

30. EGYPTIAN MYSTERIES VOL 2: Dictionary of Gods and Goddesses ISBN: 1-884564-23-2 $21.95 This book is about the mystery of neteru, the gods and goddesses of Ancient Egypt (Kamit, Kemet). Neteru means "Gods and Goddesses." But the Neterian teaching of Neteru represents more than the usual limited modern day concept of "divinities" or "spirits." The Neteru of Kamit are also metaphors, cosmic principles and vehicles for the enlightening teachings of Shetaut Neter (Ancient Egyptian-African Religion). Actually they are the elements for one of the most advanced systems of spirituality ever conceived in human history. Understanding the concept of neteru provides a firm basis for spiritual evolution and the pathway for viable culture, peace on earth and a healthy human society.   Why is it important to have gods and goddesses in our lives? In order for spiritual evolution to be possible, once a human being has accepted that there is existence after death and there is a transcendental being who exists beyond time and space knowledge, human beings need a connection to that which transcends the ordinary experience of human life in time and space and a means to understand the transcendental reality beyond the mundane reality.

31. EGYPTIAN MYSTERIES VOL. 3 The Priests and Priestesses of Ancient Egypt ISBN: 1-884564-53-4 $22.95 This volume details the path of Neterian priesthood, the joys, challenges and rewards of advanced Neterian life, the teachings that allowed the priests and priestesses to manage the most long lived civilization in human history and how that path can be adopted today; for those who want to tread the path of the Clergy of Shetaut Neter.

32. THE KING OF EGYPT: The Struggle of Good and Evil for Control of the World and The Human Soul ISBN 1-8840564-44-5 $18.95 This volume contains a novelized version of the Asarian Resurrection myth that is based on the actual scriptures presented in the Book Asarian Religion (old name –Resurrecting Osiris). This volume is prepared in the form of a screenplay and can be easily adapted to be used as a stage play. Spiritual seeking is a mythic journey that has many emotional highs and lows, ecstasies and depressions, victories and frustrations. This is the War of Life that is played out in the myth as the struggle of Heru and Set and those are mythic characters that represent the human Higher and Lower self. How to understand the war and emerge victorious in the journey o life? The ultimate victory and fulfillment can be experienced, which is not changeable or lost in time. The purpose of myth is to convey the wisdom of life through the story of divinities who show the way to overcome the challenges and foibles of life. In this volume the feelings and emotions of the characters of the myth have been highlighted to show the deeply rich texture of the Ancient Egyptian myth. This myth contains deep spiritual teachings and insights into the nature of self, of God and the mysteries of life and the means to discover the true meaning of life and thereby achieve the true purpose of life. To become victorious in the battle of life means to become the King (or Queen) of Egypt.Have you seen movies like The Lion King, Hamlet, The Odyssey, or The Little Buddha? These have been some of the most popular movies in modern times. The Sema Institute of Yoga is dedicated to researching and presenting the wisdom and culture of ancient Africa. The Script is designed to be produced as a motion picture but may be addapted for the theater as well. $19.95   copyright 1998 By Dr. Muata Ashby

33.   AFRICAN DIONYSUS: FROM EGYPT TO GREECE: The Kamitan Origins of Greek Culture and Religion ISBN: 1-884564-47-X $24.95 U.S. FROM EGYPT TO GREECE This insightful manual is a reference to Ancient Egyptian mythology and philosophy and its correlation to what later became known as Greek and Rome mythology and philosophy. It outlines the basic tenets of the mythologies and shoes the ancient origins of Greek culture in Ancient Egypt. This volume also documents the origins of the Greek alphabet in Egypt as well as Greek religion, myth and philosophy of the gods and goddesses from Egypt from the myth of Atlantis and archaic period with the Minoans to the Classical period. This volume also acts as a resource for Colleges students who would like to set up fraternities and sororities based on the original Ancient Egyptian principles of Sheti and Maat philosophy. ISBN: 1-884564-47-X $22.95 U.S.

34.   THE FORTY TWO PRECEPTS OF MAAT, THE PHILOSOPHY OF RIGHTEOUS ACTION AND THE ANCIENT EGYPTIAN WISDOM TEXTS <u>ADVANCED STUDIES</u> This manual is designed for use with the 1998 Maat Philosophy Class conducted by Dr. Muata Ashby. This is a detailed study of Maat Philosophy. It contains a compilation of the 42 laws or precepts of Maat and the corresponding principles which they represent along with the teachings of the ancient Egyptian Sages relating to each. Maat philosophy was the basis of Ancient Egyptian society and government as well as the heart of Ancient Egyptian myth and spirituality. Maat is at once a goddess, a cosmic force and a living social doctrine, which promotes social harmony and thereby paves the way for spiritual evolution in all levels of society. ISBN: 1-884564-48-8 $16.95 U.S.

Music Based on the Prt M Hru and other Kemetic Texts

Available on Compact Disc $14.99 and Audio Cassette $9.99

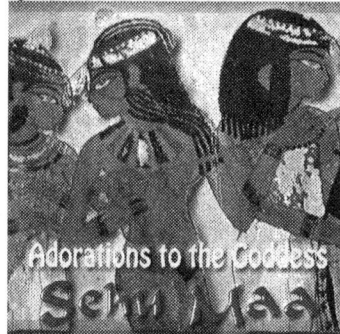

Adorations to the Goddess

Music for Worship of the Goddess

NEW Egyptian Yoga Music CD
by Sehu Maa
Ancient Egyptian Music CD
Instrumental Music played on reproductions of Ancient Egyptian Instruments– Ideal for meditation and
reflection on the Divine and for the practice of spiritual programs and Yoga exercise sessions.

©1999 By Muata Ashby
CD $14.99 –

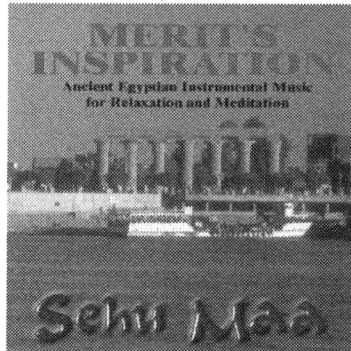

MERIT'S INSPIRATION
NEW Egyptian Yoga Music CD
by Sehu Maa
Ancient Egyptian Music CD
Instrumental Music played on
reproductions of Ancient Egyptian Instruments– Ideal for meditation and
reflection on the Divine and for the practice of spiritual programs and Yoga exercise sessions.
©1999 By
Muata Ashby
CD $14.99 –
UPC# 761527100429

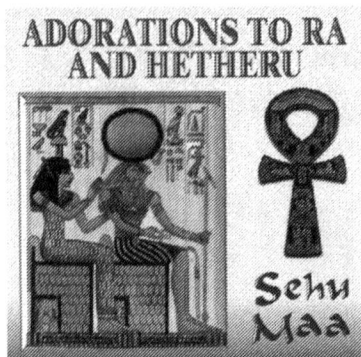

ANORATIONS TO RA AND HETHERU
NEW Egyptian Yoga Music CD
By Sehu Maa (Muata Ashby)
Based on the Words of Power of Ra and HetHeru
played on reproductions of Ancient Egyptian Instruments **Ancient Egyptian Instruments used: Voice, Clapping, Nefer Lute, Tar Drum, Sistrums, Cymbals** – The Chants, Devotions, Rhythms and Festive Songs Of the Neteru – Ideal for meditation, and devotional singing and dancing.

©1999 By Muata Ashby
CD $14.99 –
UPC# 761527100221

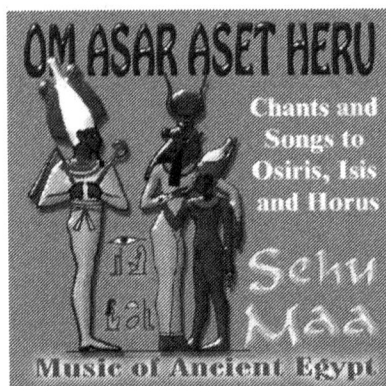

SONGS TO ASAR ASET AND HERU
NEW
Egyptian Yoga Music CD
By Sehu Maa
played on reproductions of Ancient Egyptian Instruments– The Chants, Devotions, Rhythms and Festive Songs Of the Neteru - Ideal for meditation, and devotional singing and dancing.
Based on the Words of Power of Asar (Asar), Aset (Aset) and Heru (Heru) Om Asar Aset Heru is the third in a series of musical explorations of the Kemetic (Ancient Egyptian) tradition of music. Its ideas are based on the Ancient Egyptian Religion of Asar, Aset and Heru and it is designed for listening, meditation and worship. ©1999 By Muata Ashby
CD $14.99 –
UPC# 761527100122

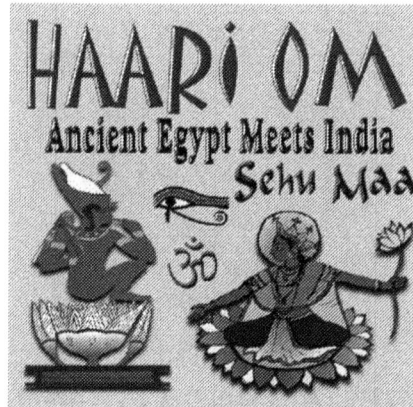

HAARI OM: ANCIENT EGYPT MEETS INDIA IN MUSIC
NEW Music CD
By Sehu Maa

The Chants, Devotions, Rhythms and
Festive Songs Of the Ancient Egypt and India, harmonized and played on reproductions of ancient instruments along with modern instruments and beats. Ideal for meditation, and devotional singing and dancing.
Haari Om is the fourth in a series of musical explorations of the Kemetic (Ancient Egyptian) and Indian traditions of music, chanting and devotional spiritual practice. Its ideas are based on the Ancient Egyptian Yoga spirituality and Indian Yoga spirituality.
©1999 By Muata Ashby
CD $14.99 –
UPC# 761527100528

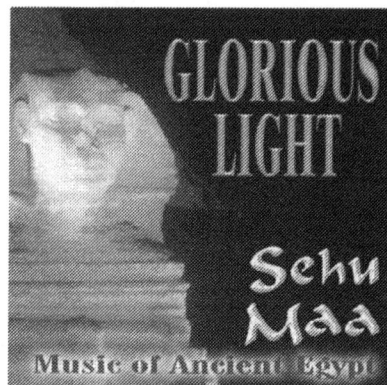

RA AKHU: THE GLORIOUS LIGHT
NEW
Egyptian Yoga Music CD
By Sehu Maa

The fifth collection of original music compositions based on the Teachings and Words of The Trinity, the God Asar and the Goddess Nebethet, the Divinity Aten, the God Heru, and the Special Meditation Hekau or Words of Power of Ra from the Ancient Egyptian Tomb of Seti I and more...
played on reproductions of Ancient Egyptian Instruments and modern instruments - Ancient Egyptian Instruments used: Voice, Clapping, Nefer Lute, Tar Drum, Sistrums, Cymbals
— The Chants, Devotions, Rhythms and Festive Songs Of the Neteru – Ideal for meditation, and devotional singing and dancing.
©1999 By Muata Ashby
CD $14.99 –
UPC# 761527100825

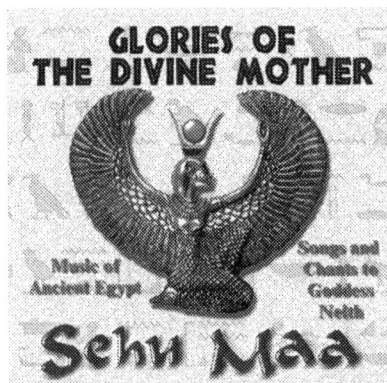

GLORIES OF THE DIVINE MOTHER
Based on the hieroglyphic text of the worship of Goddess Net.
The Glories of The Great Mother
©2000 Muata Ashby
CD $14.99 UPC# 761527101129`

Order Form

Telephone orders: Call Toll Free: 1(305) 378-6253. Have your AMEX, Optima, Visa or MasterCard ready.

Fax orders: 1-(305) 378-6253   E-MAIL ADDRESS: Semayoga@aol.com

Postal Orders: Sema Institute of Yoga, P.O. Box 570459, Miami, Fl. 33257. USA.

Please send the following books and / or tapes.

ITEM

_____Cost $_____

_____Cost $_____

_____Cost $_____

_____Cost $_____

_____Cost $_____

Total $_____

Name:_____

Physical Address:_____

City:_____ State:_____ Zip:_____

Sales tax: Please add 6.5% for books shipped to Florida addresses

_____Shipping: $6.50 for first book and .50¢ for each additional

_____Shipping: Outside US $5.00 for first book and $3.00 for each additional

_____Payment:_____

_____Check -Include Driver License #:

_____

_____Credit card: _____ Visa, _____ MasterCard, _____ Optima,
_____ AMEX.

Card number:_____

Name on card:_____ Exp. date:_____/_____

www.ingramcontent.com/pod-product-compliance
Lightning Source LLC
Chambersburg PA
CBHW080250030426
42334CB00023BA/2770